THE A-Z
OF HOMŒOPATHY

THE A-Z
OF HOMŒOPATHY

by Trevor M. Cook
M. Sc., Ph.D. (Lond), C. Eng., M I Prod. E., C. Chem., FRSC.

W. Foulsham & Co. Ltd.
London • New York • Toronto • Cape Town • Sydney

W. Foulsham & Company Limited
Yeovil Road, Slough, Berkshire, SL1 4JH

ISBN 0-572-01311-6

Printed in Great Britain
at The Bath Press, Avon

4

This book is dedicated to my family
for their unfailing support and encouragement.

Contents

List of Illustrations

Plant Illustrations by Jason Adamson

Preface

Homœopathy, like every field of medicine and science has created its own vocabulary and uses it to explain its concepts. Some words are entirely new and specific to homœopathy, whilst others are common words which used in the context of homœopathy take on a whole new meaning. The word Homœopathy itself was coined by Samuel Hahnemann, its founder, from two Greek words *homoios* (like or similar) and *pathos* (suffering).

In recent years homœopathy has been receiving increasing public support. More and more people are wishing to learn about homœopathy and seeking homœopathic treatment. Those who are new to homœopathy encounter many of these words which are unfamiliar and this can cause confusion or reduce their understanding of the subject.

This book, which serves as a supplement to the textbooks or a day-to-day reference book, sets out key words commonly used in homœopathic literature in an alphabetical list, each with a simple definition. Fifty homœopathic remedies which are frequently prescribed are also listed and many of the leading contributors to the progress of homœopathy in the past are included. Where possible, cross references are given.

The index of homœopathic terms includes the most common homœopathic medicines. It is primarily intended to assist doctors, practitioners, nurses, veterinary surgeons, pharmacists and lay people involved in self-help programmes. It should also prove useful to those already receiving homœopathic treatment who wish to learn more about this safe and effective therapy.

The main index is followed by a comprehensive alphabetical list of homœopathic medicines, an index of common abbreviations used in homœopathy and a list of the top fifty homœopathic medicines and their uses. A recommended reading list and addresses of national organisations, who would be pleased to assist the reader, are also included.

I would like to record my grateful thanks to my wife Barbara, and to my family for their advice and encouragement, to Garth and Mary Young, and to so many homœopaths, too numerous to mention individually, whose kindness and friendship have sustained me.

London 1985   *Dr. Trevor M. Cook*

A to Z of Homœopathy

A

ABBREVIATIONS
For index of abbreviations see page 63.

ACONITUM NAPELLUS
Aconite. Monk's hood. Monkshood. Wolfsbane.
Member of the Ranunculaceæ family. Tall plant with flowers
shaped like a monk's cowl, growing in mountainous areas. Plant
contains the very poisonous alkaloid, aconitine. The mother
tincture is prepared from the whole plant.

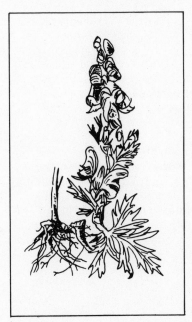

1. Aconitum napellus

Short–acting remedy valuable at early stages of acute
conditions, for example colds of influenza. Treatment of effects
of fear and fright, sore throat, croup, chicken pox and facial
neuralgia related to cold. Symptoms are worse about midnight,

worsened by dry, cold winds, and improved by perspiration. Veterinary uses include the early treatment of distemper.

ACTÆA RACEMOSA
Actæa rac. Baneberry. Herb Christopher. Homœopathic remedy with an affinity for the musculo-skeletal system and female sexual system. The mother tincture is prepared from the root of the plant. Used mainly for the treatment of neuralgia, stiff neck, headaches, effects of over-exertion or fright, change of life. Symptoms are improved by warmth and worse in the morning, in the cold and damp, and from movement.

ACUTE DISEASE
Having a rapid onset, a short duration and pronounced symptoms (cf. *Chronic Disease*). The term does not indicate the severity of a disease.

ADDICTION
Homœopathic remedies are non-addictive in all dosages.

ADELAIDE, Queen
Wife and Consort of King William IV, who introduced homœopathy into the British Royal Family in 1835. Queen Adelaide began a tradition of Royal support for homœopathy spanning six generations to the present day.
See *Royal Patronage*.

ADMINISTRATION of Homœopathic Medicines
Pilules or tablets are best taken, dry and untouched by hand, under the tongue. It is preferable to rinse the mouth with water if food has recently been eaten or if toothpaste has just been used. The medicine is usually administered on rising in the morning or retiring at night, but in any case away from food. Some homœopathic doctors advise that coffee should be avoided during treatment. Alcoholic drinks should be avoided, but a little wine may be permissible.
See *Frequency of Dosage*.

AGGRAVATION
A temporary or transient worsening of symptoms sometimes resulting from the taking of a homœopathic medicine, usually followed by a rapid improvement in the patient's condition. The sign > is used to indicate an aggravation.
See *Law of Similars*; *Modalities*.

ALLIUM CEPA
Cepa. Onion. Common Red Onion.
Like veratrum album and colchicum autumale, allium cepa is a member of the Liliaceæ family. Native of Western Asia, it is cultivated throughout Europe. The mother tincture is prepared from the whole fresh plant gathered in July or August.
Used extensively for the treatment of common colds with much sneezing and watering of the eyes and hacking coughs, particularly those worsened by cold air.

ALLOPATHY
A word coined by Samuel Hahnemann (q.v.) to describe conventional or orthodox medical treatment as opposed to homœopathy. Derived from the Greek word *allos* – other, and *pathos* – suffering; thus 'other suffering'. The treatment of disease by an unrelated substance to induce a different tendency to suppress the symptoms in contrast to homœopathy.

ALTERNATIVE MEDICINE
Alternatives to allopathic (q.v.) or conventional medical treatment. These alternative therapies include homœopathy, herbalism, osteopathy, acupuncture, and chiropractic. Nowadays, the term *complementary medicine* is preferred since homœopathy is now seen as a treatment which can be used as a complement to or in conjunction with conventional therapy.

AMELIORATIONS
See *Modalities*.

ANTIBIOTICS
Substances produced by living micro-organisms (eg. mould or bacteria) with antimicrobial therapeutic properties; for example, tetracycline, penicillinum calcium, penicillum notatum. Used homœopathically only in potencies.

ANTIPATHIC MEDICINE
Conventional (or allopathic q.v.) medicine.

ANTIPATHY
The treatment by opposites to neutralise a disease symptom.

APIS MELLIFICA
Apis mel. Honey bee.
The mother tincture is prepared from the whole bee.
A useful homœopathic remedy, mainly for the treatment of

burning, stinging pains, sunburn, swelling of lower eyelids, abscesses, swollen ankles and insect stings. Symptoms are improved by cold.

ARNDT–SCHULTZ LAW

The inversion of the effects of a drug as a function of the dose. This law states that small doses of drugs (i.e. in potencies) encourage life activity, large material doses impede life activity and very large doses destroy life activity.
See *Dosage*.

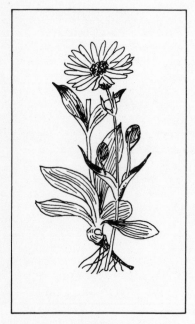

2. Arnica montana

ARNICA MONTANA

Arnica. Mountain Arnica. Leopard's Bane. Panacea Lapsorum. Alpine flower, normally grown at an altitude of 3,500 feet.
A very common, effective homœopathic remedy used mainly for the treatment after injuries, bruising, mental and physical shock, exhaustion and contusions. Useful before or after surgery or visits to the dentist. Symptoms are worsened by the slightest contact, by motion, and cold and damp. Symptoms are improved when lying down.

ARGENTUM NITRICUM

Argent Nit. Silver Nitrate. Formula: Ag NO_3. Mineral salt

forming soluble transparent, colourless, rhombic crystals.
Indicated for nervous, impulsive, irritable people who fear
future uncertainties. Principally used for the treatment of
headache, dyspepsia, acidity, chronic laryngitis, mental strain
and illness through overwork. A useful remedy before an
interview for a job or making a speech. Symptoms are worsened
by warmth, sweet food, worry, or overwork, and better for rest.

ARSENICUM ALBUM
Arsen Alb. Arsenicum trioxide. Arseneous Oxide. Formula: $As_2 O_3$.
Insoluble, tasteless, white powder in its pure form.
Used mainly for the treatment of stomach upsets from food
poisoning, diarrhœa, vomiting and hay fever. Digestive
conditions are associated with burning pain and intense thirst.
Symptoms are better for heat or change in position.

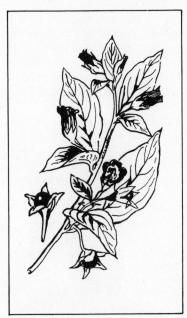

3. Atropa belladonna

ATROPA BELLADONNA
Belladonna. Deadly Nightshade.
Member of the Solanceæ family, found throughout Europe
particularly in southern England. A perennial with a hairy stem
with dull, dark green leaves, growing near hedges. Its large,
shiny, black berries are sweetish to the taste and very
poisonous. Its name is derived from 'beautiful lady' following

the use of the juice from its berries by women during the Italian Renaissance from the 14th century to beautify their eyelids. The principal constituent of the leaves is the alkaloid, atropine, which stimulates the central nervous system. The mother tincture is prepared from the whole plant, at the commencement of flowering.

A major homœopathic remedy for the treatment of sore throat, **throbbing** headache or earache, facial neuralgia, hot flushed face, chicken pox, measles, mumps and spasms. Symptoms are worsened by cold, noise, light and sudden movement and improved by rest and warmth.

Veterinary uses include swine dysentery.

ATTENUATIONS
Homœopathic dilutions. See *Potency*.

AVOGADRO'S HYPOTHESIS
The Italian physicist, Avogadro (1811) postulated that there are equal numbers of molecules or atoms in equal volumes, and the number of molecules or atoms of a substance in a unit volume has been determined by a variety of methods. From this it follows that the serial or sequential dilution of mother tinctures involved in the preparation of potencies eventually exceeds the Avogadro limit, whereby theoretically there are none of the original molecules or atoms of the starting material present in the potencies. In practice, this limit applies to potencies of 24x, 12c or higher potencies. Deviations to Avogadro's law have, however, been found experimentally and both chemical and physical differences have been observed between very high liquid potencies and pure alcohol/water solutions, indicating that the 'imprint' of the original substance has been retained. An enormous rift occurred in the late 19th century, between those physicians who favoured prescribing at potencies below and those prescribing above the Avogadro limit. See *Hughes, Dr. Richard; Kent, Dr. James*.

B

BACH REMEDIES
A range of 38 natural remedies derived from wild flowers. Additionally, there is Rescue Remedy for the treatment of shock. The remedies were developed by the late Dr. Edward Bach. Although they are essentially not homœopathic, since

they are not prepared in potencies, many people regard them as complementary.

BATCH NUMBER
Lot Number. A number used to identify each container of homœopathic medicine prepared by a licensed manufacturer. This number, which is printed on the label, enables the manufacturer to refer to records which show a complete history of the sources of materials, methods of preparation, etc.

BELLADONNA
See *Atropa Belladonna*.

BENJAMIN, Dr. Alvar (1884-1975)
Prominent homœopathic physician, who graduated as Doctor of Medicine at Sydney University. Founded The Hahnemann Society in 1958, supported by physicians and lay people who shared his concern about modern drug abuse and the use of animals in testing them.

BERBERIS
Berberis vulgaris or Berberis aquifolium. Barberry. Members of the Berberidaceæ family. Densely branched erect shrub with three-pronged needle-like spines. Grows in hedges and rocky banks. Potencies are chiefly used for treatment of renal colic. Particularly suited to intellectual people who show anxiety or fear with depression. Symptoms are not improved either by rest or exercise.

BIOCHEMIC REMEDIES
A system of medicine devised by a German physician, Dr. Schussler, based on the theory that all disease is due to a deficiency of one or more mineral salts. Twelve of these salts, known as the Schussler Salts or the *Tissue Salts*, are prepared homœopathically as triturated tablets (6x). They are: calcium fluoride, calcium phosphate, calcium sulphate, iron phosphate, magnesium phosphate, potassium phosphate, potassium chloride, potassium sulphate, sodium chloride, sodium phosphate and silicic oxide (silicea).

BLACK TYPE SYMPTOMS
Predominant symptoms. See *Repertory*.

BLACKIE, Dr. Margery Grace. C.V.O. (1898-1981)
Born at Redbourn in February 1898, she qualified as an M.D.

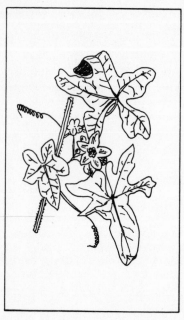

4. Bryonia dioica

at the University of London in 1928. Her first post was
Assistant Physician to the Children's Dept. of The Royal
London Homœopathic Hospital. Homœopathic physician to
H.M. The Queen – the first woman to be given this position –
from 1969 until shortly before her death in August 1981. Author
of *The Patient, Not The Cure*. Whilst Dean of the Faculty of
Homœopathy, Dr. Blackie re-introduced the training courses for
doctors. Her treatment was characterised by the prescribing of
high potencies of a single medicine. She received the order of
the C.V.O. in 1979.

BOYD, Dr. William Ernest

An outstanding homœopathic physician who graduated at the
University of Glasgow. Consultant physician to the Glasgow
Homœopathic Hospital and author of many articles, he died in
1955.

BRITISH HOMŒOPATHIC ASSOCIATION

A registered charity, the Association was founded in 1902.
Membership is open to professional people, but it is primarily
an Association for the layman. Its objectives are to spread the
knowledge and use of homœopathy and generally further the
cause of homœopathy.

The Association publishes a bi-monthly journal, Homœopathy, and maintains a library.

BRYONIA

White Bryony. Bryonia alba. Bryonia dioica.

A climbing hedgerow plant with long spiralling unbranched tendrils, growing in thickets, hedges and rocky places. There are 22 varieties of Bryonia alba and Bryonia dioica, which have the same therapeutic action. The former is found only on the continent of Europe, whilst the latter is also found in Great Britain. Bryonia alba was one of the original remedies proved by Samuel Hahnemann. The mother tincture is prepared from the root of the plant.

Potencies are widely used for the treatment of chesty colds, dry cough and muscular pains which are better after rest and congestive headache with sensation of pressure. Symptoms are worsened by movement and heat, and lessened by firm pressure at site of pain.

C

CALCAREA CARBONICA

Calc. Carb. Calcium Carbonate. Carbonate of lime. Calcarea Ostrearum.

Insoluble, white powder. Formula: $Ca CO_3$. Samuel Hahnemann chose the ground, middle layer of the oyster shell as the source for this common, polycrest remedy. Used, inter alia, for the treatment of profuse periods in young girls, acne rosacea and cramp. Sensitive, shy, easily embarrassed people are most likely to benefit. Symptoms are better for warmth and dry weather and worse for cold and damp, at night or from standing.

CALCAREA FLUORICA

Calc. Fluor. Fluorspar. Fluorite. Fluoride of lime. Calcium Fluoride. Formula: $Ca F_2$.

Naturally occurring mineral salt. Soluble, white powder or cubic crystals.

A useful remedy for the treatment of cracked joints, varicose veins, bleeding and protruding piles and thick catarrh. Used extensively to prevent tooth decay. Symptoms are better after gentle movement and worse in damp weather or after rest.

CALCAREA PHOSPHORICA

Calc. Phos. Phosphate of lime. Calcium phosphate. Insoluble white powder. Formula: $Ca_3 (PO_4)_2$.

Used mainly for the treatment of severe stomach pains after eating, slow healing fractures, brainfag, general debility associated with chronic joint conditions and acne. Symptoms are worse for a change in weather conditions.

CALENDULA OFFICINALIS

Calendula. Common Marigold. Pot marigold. Gold Bloom. Mary-bud.

Probably a native plant of the Mediterranean region. Spreading annual with solitary orange – yellow flower. The mother tincture is freshly prepared from the whole flowering plant.

An effective healing agent taken internally usually in 6th centesimal potency or locally as ointment or cream, as a healing agent for open wounds and sores. A basic first aid treatment.

Most beneficial for depressed, easily frightened, irritable people.

CANTHARIS

Spanish fly. Blister beetle.

Small, brilliant blue-green beetle, about 2 cm (1 in) in length. Strong odour with pungent taste. The mother tincture is prepared from the dried, powdered insect.

Used principally for acute, irritating conditions of the mucous membrane, for example, the treatment of burning pains in the bladder before and after passing water, and for burns and scalds before the formation of blisters, sunburn and cystitis. Symptoms are better for warm applications and worse for drinking (especially water) and whilst urinating.

CARBO VEGETABILIS

Carbo Veg. Vegetable Charcoal. Black Charcoal.

Residue from the controlled burning of beech or birch wood, as amorphous black carbon with traces of mineral salts. Lower potencies are prepared by trituration (q.v.). Exhibits certain affinities with various body tissues.

Used principally for the treatment of indigestion with excessive flatulence, hoarseness, collapse, debility and acne. Patients with dislike of darkness, embarrassed in company or prone to sudden loss of memory are most likely to benefit. Symptoms are worse for cold air and overwork.

CENTESIMAL POTENCY

See *Potency*.

CHAMOMILLA

Wild Chamomile. German Chamomile.
Annual herb with large, fibrous root; 30-60 cm (1-2 ft) high
erect stem with slender branches. Member of the compositæ
family. Flowers are white florets, blooming from May to
August. Grows throughout Europe to Northern Asia and India.
Its chemical constituents include potassium, calcium, glucose
and gallic acid. The mother tincture is prepared from the whole
plant. One of the original 26 remedies listed by Samuel
Hahnemann in part two of his book, *Fragmenta di viribus
Medicamentorum positivus sive in sano capore humano observatis*,
published 1805.

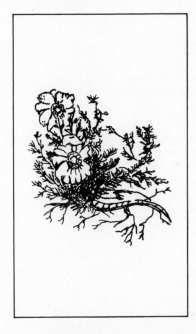

5. Chamomilla

Used extensively in granular form for fractious and teething
infants and for the relief of nausea, migraine and bladder pain
and mothers with nursing problems. Symptoms are worsened by
anger and improved by heat. Improvement in the infant when
held in the arms or walked about. In Samuel Hahnemann's
own words, Chamomilla is especially suited to the child *'which
makes itself stiff and bends backwards, stamps with its feet on the nurse's
arm. Cries in an uncontrollable way, wants this thing and the other and
when given anything it is refused or knocked away'*.

CHROMATOGRAPHY
A laboratory technique for separating and identifying constituents of liquid or gaseous mixtures. **Thin Layer Chromatography** has found a particular application with homœopathic mother tinctures, whereby characteristic bands representing their individual chemical constituents are produced on a specially prepared plate coated with an inert material. See *Quality Control*.

CHRONIC DISEASE
A deep seated disease of long duration with symptoms which are constantly present or recurring (see *Acute Disease*). Chronic diseases are therefore more difficult to treat successfully, particularly homœopathically, since it aims to effect a fundamental, complete cure and not simply act as a palliative.

CHRONIC DISEASES, THE
Title of major work by Dr. Samuel Hahnemann, originally published in 1828 as *The Chronic Diseases, Their Peculiar Nature and Their Homœopathic Cure*.

COMBINATION REMEDIES
Combinations of two or more homœopathic remedies used simultaneously in a course of treatment. Hahnemann advocated the use of a single remedy only at any time, and the use of combination remedies has, therefore, given rise to some controversy. However, the efficacy of certain combination remedies has been demonstrated, particularly with the polycrests (q.v.).

CINCHONA
China. Peruvian Bark. Cortex peruvianus.
Prepared from the bark of the quinaquina tree which grows on the eastern slopes of the Andes. Contains mainly alkaloids, principally quinine. Used for centuries for the treatment of malaria after it had been brought to Europe by missionaries in South America. Named by Linnæus from the Duchess of Cinchon, Vice-Queen of Peru who was cured by the drug. The subject of Samuel Hahnemann's original proving (q.v.) of a remedy, whilst translating, in 1790, *A Treatise on Materia Medica* by Dr. William Cullen when he experienced symptoms similar to malaria, the disease the drug was used to treat.
Hahnemann's observations foreshadowed his enunciation of the basic principle of homœopathy in 1796.

Used for hæmostatic treatment, treatment during convalescence and digestive disorders. Symptoms are worsened by draughts or light pressure and improved by heat. Often considered for dehydrated patients after illness.

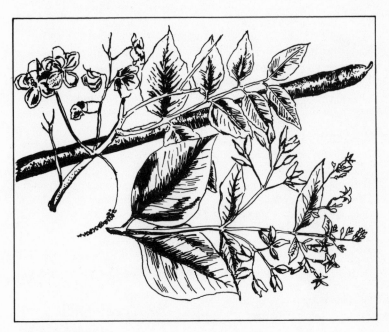

6. Cinchona

CLINICAL TRIALS

The testing of medicines or drugs to prove their efficacy in the treatment of humans and animals. Conventional medicines are tested according to procedures laid down by the Department of Health (based on the so called 'double blind' technique), in order to gain product licences (q.v.) under the Medicines Act 1968 and 1971. Clinical trials of homœopathic medicines by these conventional procedures are not entirely appropriate because of their patient-orientated prescribing. Furthermore, it is difficult for the relatively small number of homœopaths to collect sufficient numbers of patients and there is a long follow-up to assess the benefits accurately.

One of the earliest successful homœopathic clinical trials was carried out during the second World War on the prevention and treatment of mustard gas burns (Paterson 1944).

COCCULUS INDICUS
Anamirta cocculus. Levant nut. Indian cockle. Fish berry. Climbing plant with yellow flowers and heartshaped leaves, indigenous to India and Sri Lanka.
Valuable treatment for travel sickness, nausea with a hollow sensation in the stomach and nausea during pregnancy and bodily and mental strain. Suited to people who are apprehensive and unable to make decisions. Symptoms are worse on drinking or eating or lack of sleep.

COLCHICUM
Colchicum autumnale. Autumn crocus. Meadow Saffron. Naked Maiden.
Like veratrum album it is a member of the Liliaceæ family. Grows from a large corm, 3.5 cm ($1\frac{1}{2}$ ins) in diameter, in damp meadows. White or pale rose flower. The mother tincture is prepared from the juice of the fresh corm lifted in March or April. Main constituent is the alkaloid, colchicine.
Used essentially in acute conditions, especially when the patient is weak and extremely sensitive and irritable. Useful for gout.

COMPLEMENTARY MEDICINE
See *Alternative Medicine*.

CONSTITUTIONAL REMEDY
A remedy prescribed according to the temperament, character and general disposition of the patient, in addition to the symptoms of the disease. Hence 'constitutional type'. For example, the 'Pulsatilla type' is the weepy blonde, whilst the 'Arnica type' wants solitude and cannot bear being touched.

CONTAINERS
Traditionally, pure glass containers have been used for homœopathic medicines since it is inert and impermeable. Although plastic containers are generally satisfactory, laboratory tests have shown that some types of plastic in contact with an alcohol and water mixture produce modifications in the ultra-violet absorption spectrum after two hours, indicating that some plastics may affect the ingredients contained in them.

C POTENCIES

Centesimal series of potencies (q.v.) derived from dilutions or attenuations of mother tinctures in the ratio of 1:100. See *Potencies*; *Dilutions*.

CUPRUM METALLICUM

Cuprum Met. Metallic copper.
Reddish, lustrous metal. Symbol: Cu. Potencies are prepared by trituration of the powdered metal:
Useful remedy for the treatment of cramp in extremities, nausea with stomach pain, poor circulation and whooping cough.

D

DEADLY NIGHTSHADE

See *Atropa belladonna*.

DECIMAL POTENCY

See *Potency*.

DILUTIONS (HOMŒOPATHIC)

There are two series designating the degree of dilution of mother tinctures; one based on dilutions in 10's and the other based on dilutions in 100's. Thus, we have:

Decimal Series

1x	1 part in 10 parts	1 : 10	10^{-1}
2x	1 part in 100 parts	1 : 100	10^{-2}
3x	1 part in 1,000 parts	1 : 1,000	10^{-3}
6x	1 part in 1,000,000 parts	1 : 1,000,000	10^{-6}
12x	1 part in 1,000,000,000,000	1 : 1,000,000,000,000	10^{-12}
30x			10^{-30}

Centesimal Series

1(c)	1 part in 100	1 : 100	10^{-2}
2(c)	1 part in 10,000	1 : 10,000	10^{-4}
3(c)	1 part in 1,000,000	1 : 1,000,000	10^{-6}
6(c)	1 part in 1,000,000,000,000	1 : 1,000,000,000,000	10^{-12}
30(c)			10^{-60}
200(c)			10^{-400}

See *Potency*.

DISEASE PICTURE

The totality of the symptoms of an illness. These are matched with the drug picture (q.v.) in homœopathic prescribing.

DOSAGE

The prescribed frequency and quantity of a medicine to be taken at one time. A single dose is described as a unit dose. The frequency of the dose is more important in homœopathic treatment than the quantity of the infinitesimally small doses involved. It is fundamental not to repeat a dosage when an improvement in the patient's condition is apparent.
Homœopathy is more a qualitative rather than a quantitative therapy so the correct selection of the remedy is of prime importance. Although important, potency and dosage are secondary considerations. See *Frequency of Dose*.

DRAMATIC DISEASE

See *Acute Disease*.

DROSERA ROTUNDIFOLIA

Drosera. Sundew. Moor grass. Red Rot.
Small plant with reddish circular leaves which grows all over Europe in peat bogs and damp heathland. The mother tincture is prepared from the whole plant.
Its action on the upper respiratory tract finds use in the treatment of persistent, tickling, irritating coughs with retching and vomiting and whooping cough.

DRUG PICTURE

A summary of the symptoms, mental states and pathological changes that a medicinal substance is capable of *causing* and thereby treating the patient according to the basic homœopathic principle.

DYNAMISATION

The release of latent energy of natural substances in the preparation of homœopathic medicines by means of trituration or in the case of fluids, by serial dilution followed by succussion at each step. (Hahnemann, *The Chronic Diseases*)
See *Potency. Potentisation*.

E

EUPHRASIA OFFICIANALIS
Euphrasia. Eyebright.
Member of the Scrophulariaceæ family. Occurs throughout
Europe in meadows and open woods in about fifty sub-species.
The mother tincture is prepared from the whole plant.
Used principally for the treatment of inflamed, burning or
watering eyes, streaming nose, conjunctivitis, hayfever and early
stages of measles or German measles. The patient may have no
desire to converse. He or she may be indolent or depressed.
Symptoms are worse from wind, light and at night and better
from cold washing and daylight.

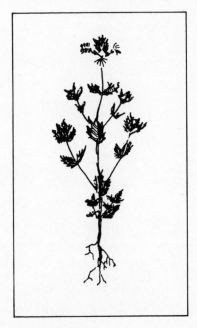

7. Euphrasia officinalis

EXCIPIENT
A material in which the active ingredient in the form of the
potentised homœopathic medicine is incorporated. For example,
lactose (q.v.).

F

FACULTY OF HOMŒOPATHY

Originally known as the British Homœopathic Society on its formation by Dr. Frederick Harvey Foster Quin (q.v.) in 1844. It became the Faculty of Homœopathy in 1943, and powers were conferred on its members by the Faculty of Homœopathy Act 1950.

The Faculty aims to advance the principles and to extend the practice of homœopathy. Meeting in the Royal London Homœopathic Hospital and in the provinces, the Faculty conducts postgraduate teaching in homœopathic medicine and publishes *The British Homœopathic Journal* quarterly.

Associateship of the Faculty is open to doctors on the Register of the General Medical Council and to dentists, veterinary surgeons, pharmacists and state registered nurses.

FERRUM PHOSPHORICUM

Ferr. Phos. Iron phosphate. Ferric Phosphate.

Brown powder, Formula: $Fe\ PO_4$.

Naturally occurring mineral salt, as beraunite, cacoxenite or dufrenite.

Used in potencies for the treatment of inter alia; fear, variable appetite, nose bleed, coughs and colds with anæmia and recurrent middle ear infections.

See also *Biochemic Remedies*.

FIRST AID

Homœopathy is most effective in the treatment of accidents, injuries and shock. Principal remedies used are Aconite (mental or physical shock), Calendula (cuts and abrasions), Arnica (bruises and sprains), Hypericum (nerve injuries – splinter wounds, bites, crushed fingers or toes), Ledum (pierced skin) and Rhus Tox (strains), Ruta Grav (strained ligaments), Urtica Urens (nettle stings) and Pyrethrum (insect bites and stings).

FLUXION

A special method of homœopathic potentisation, sometimes used for the preparation of very high potencies, for example; 50M, CM.

FREQUENCY of Dosage

Generally, for acute conditions, homœopathic medicines are given more frequently than for chronic conditions. Further, lower potencies are given more frequently than higher potencies. The duration of action of the medicine in the body may also vary with different medicines. As a general rule however, the frequency of dose should be every 2 to 4 hours for acute conditions and twice a day for 2 to 3 days, or perhaps only 3 to 4 doses a week for chronic conditions.

Important note: Consult a physician in cases of serious illness. See also *Dosage* and *Administration of Homœopathic Medicines*.

G

GELSEMIUM SEMPERVIRENS

Gelsemium. Yellow Jasmine. Carolina Yasmine.

Native plant of America. Contains the alkaloids gelseminine, and gelsemine. The mother tincture is prepared from the fresh root.

An invaluable first aid homœopathic remedy and one of the polycrests (q.v.) it is used extensively in potencies for the treatment of influenza, sore throat (with a desire to drink) and runny nose, nervous anxiety and emotional states, examination

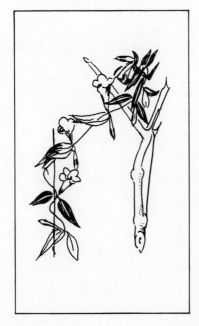

8. Gelsemium sempervirens

nerves, measles and headache and migraine. Symptoms are worsened by damp, impending storms, heat and emotion and improved by movement, open air or urination.

GENERALS
General symptoms, to which the homœopathic physician attaches great importance, affecting the whole body or personality, for example general tiredness or shivering. See *Particulars*; *Mentals*.

GLASS
See *Containers*.

GRAFTING
A variation of the Korsakov (q.v.) method of preparing liquid potencies, whereby diluent is added to a container of any liquid potency which has been emptied except for the liquid adhering to the walls. This haphazard dilution is considered thoroughly reprehensible by dedicated homœopathic pharmacists.

GRAM, Dr. H. B.
Danish doctor who introduced homœopathy into the U.S.A. in 1825.

GRANULE
A pharmaceutical form of homœopathic medicine, originally used by Hahnemann, especially suitable for administration to children and infants. Prepared from a mixture of pure sucrose and lactose, in the form of small spheres weighing about 5 centigrammes.

GRAPHITES
Black lead. Graphite. Plumbago. Mineral Carbon.
Naturally occurring element. Symbol: C. Crystallised graphite with traces of iron and silica, mainly in Canada and Sri Lanka. Samuel Hahnemann prepared the homœopathic medicine from the 'purest black lead of a fine English pencil'.
Used in potencies for the treatment of cracked, weeping eczema and chapped, unhealthy skin and constipation. Most likely to benefit are cautious, uncertain people, overweight or in adolescence. Symptoms are worse at night before midnight and in draughts.

H

HAEHL, Dr. Richard

Leading German homœopathic physician who practised in Stuttgart. He travelled extensively in Britain, the USA and Europe whilst researching for his best known work, a detailed biography of Dr. Samuel Hahnemann which was published in 1922. He died in 1932.

HAHNEMANN, Dr. Christian Friedrich Samuel (1755–1843)

The founder of the modern system of homœopathic medicine. Samuel Hahnemann was born in Meissen, Saxony on 10 April 1755, the second son of a porcelain artist. A gifted student, he read medicine at the University of Leipzig and, subsequently, at the University of Erlangen where he graduated as Doctor of Medicine in 1779. He soon became disenchanted with medicine as it was practised at that time and campaigned for medical reform throughout his life. He wrote numerous articles condemning inadequate and insanitary housing conditions and barbaric and cruel medical practices, such as blood–letting and the treatment of the mentally ill. He advocated proper diet, regular exercise, adequate rest and improved social conditions. Having virtually given up practising medicine, he embarked with his wife Johanna Henriette (née Kuchler), on continuous travels over many years, earning his living mainly through translating medical books (he was a brilliant linguist). He finally settled in Leipzig after the publication of his greatest work, *The Organon of the Rational Art of Healing* (q.v.) in which he enunciated the principles of homœopathy. Virtually driven out of Leipzig by the local apothecaries and physicians who were violently opposed to his safe, gentle and effective system of healing, Hahnemann moved to Köthen. In this town he practised homœopathy with great success until the death of his wife and his retirement. He continued to publish articles on homœopathy, and wrote two more major works – *Materia Medica Pura* (six parts, 1811–1821) and *The Chronic Diseases Their Peculiar Nature and Their Homœopathic Cure* (1828) (q.v.).

In 1835, Hahnemann married Melanie d'Hervilly and moved to Paris, where he started up in practice again. He died there on 3 July 1843 in his ninetieth year, having established homœopathy as a humane and natural system of medicine which was sweeping throughout the world, and to earn the gratitude of generations yet to come.

HAHNEMANNIAN

In accordance with the principles and practice of homœopathy set down by Dr. Samuel Hahnemann. For example: *Hahnemannian* potentisation.

HAHNEMANN SOCIETY

A registered charity, The Hahnemann Society was founded by Dr. Alva Benjamin in 1958. Its objectives are to educate the public in the principles of homœopathy and in its safety and efficacy in the treatment of sick people and animals. It also seeks to promote and encourage the study and practice of homœopathy. Membership is open to both professional and lay people.

The Society publishes a quarterly, illustrated magazine entitled *Homœopathy Today*, which is free to members.

HALF-HOMŒOPATH

Description used by Samuel Hahnemann in the *Leipzig Tageblatt* in 1832, to show his displeasure with homœopathic doctors who also practised allopathy (q.v.). Nowadays, allopathic medicine is seen as complementary to homœopathic medicine.

HAMAMELIS VIRGINICA

Hamamelis. Witch Hazel.

Homœopathic remedy proved by Dr. Constantine Hering (q.v.). Mother tincture, which is deep red in colour, prepared from the fresh bark of twigs or the root.

Excellent remedy for varicose veins, heavy periods, bleeding piles, bruises and chilblains. Symptoms are worse in warm, moist air, from touch and during the day. Symptoms are better outdoors.

HEPAR SUPHURIS

Hepar Sulph. Calcium Sulphide. Hepar Calcis.

White/yellowish powder, Formula: CaS. One of the original homœopathic remedies proved by Samuel Hahnemann, which he prepared by burning equal parts of finely powdered oyster shell and pure flowers of sulphur at white heat.

Used in potencies mainly for the treatment of offensive purulent conditions, boils, chronic suppurations croup, boils, and abscesses and wheezing. Useful remedy for infections of the upper respiratory tract, and liver. Patients have disposition to unsociability, and are sensitive to cold and open air. Symptoms are worse from uncovering head in dry, cold weather and better in damp weather.

HERING, Dr. Constantine (1800–1880)

One of the founders of homœopathy in America. Born in Oschatz in Saxony on 1st January 1800, he studied medicine at the Universities of Leipzig and Wuertzburg. He travelled widely in South America before settling in the United States, where he founded the American Academy of Homœopathic Healing in Allentown, Pennsylvania. He was one of the founders of the American Institute of Homœopathy and became its first President.

Dr. Hering proved many new homœopathic medicines, notably Lachesis (q.v.), Spigelia and Theridion.

HERING'S LAW

See *Hering, Dr. Constantine.* This Law states that 'Symptoms improve during homœopathic treatment from above downwards; from the most vital to the less vital organ and from the latest to the earliest symptoms.'

HETEROPATHY

Alternative name for Allopathy (q.v.).

HIPPOCRATES

Greek physician (circa 460 – 350 B.C.), generally regarded as the Father of Medicine. He was the author of a number of medical works and first suggested the principle of homœopathic cure.

HOLISTIC MEDICINE

See *Wholistic Medicine.*

HOMEOPATHY

American spelling of Homœopathy.

HOMŒOPATHY

The safe, gentle and effective system of healing enunciated by Dr. Samuel Hahnemann (q.v.) in his quintessential work, *The Organon of the Rational Art of Healing*, published in 1810.

The word Homœopathy was derived by Hahnemann from the Greek words *homoios*, meaning like or similar, and *pathos*, meaning suffering; hence 'like suffering'. This embraces the basic principle of homœopathy – the Law of Similars or the 'treatment of like with like'. Hahnemann described it thus:

'Every medicine which, among the symptoms it can cause in a healthy person, reproduces those most present in a given disease, is capable of curing the disease in the swiftest, most thorough and most enduring

fashion.' The basic principle is often expressed in the phrase: Similia Similibus Curentur – 'let like be treated by likes'. The homœopathic approach to cure is by stimulating the body's own defences against disease. Thus the symptoms of the disease, which are seen as the result of the body's recuperative powers fighting the disease, are stimulated by the smallest effective dose of a homœopathic remedy, so chosen because it induces similar symptoms.

Homœopathy aims to treat the whole person rather than the disease. The homœopathic physician builds up a multi-dimentional picture of the patient which will be matched with an appropriate drug picture derived from the proving (q.v.). Thus, different patients with the same disease may be treated with different remedies.

See *Symptoms*; *Constitutional Remedies*; *Cure*; *Law of Similars*; *Infinitesimal Dose*.

HOMOPATHY

A word used wrongly in the past by some allopathic doctors to describe homœopathy. *Homo* is from the Greek meaning 'same' as opposed to *homiois* – 'similar' – in homœopathy.

HORNBURG, Dr. Christian Gottlieb

One of Samuel Hahnemann's original team of provers of homœopathic medicines, who became a homœopathic martyr. Failed in his examinations at the University of Leipzig for his support for homœopathy, his medicines were later confiscated by the High Court. In 1831, after treating a patient homœopathically, he was charged with preventing proper treatment and sentenced to two months imprisonment. He died of a hæmorrhage three days after the verdict.

HOSPITALS

Homœopathic hospitals within the National Health Service are as follows:

The Royal London Homœopathic Hospital,
    Gt. Ormond Street, London WC1N 3HR

The Glasgow Homœopathic Hospital,
    1000 Gt. Western Road, Glasgow, G12 ORN
    Outpatients Department, 5 Lynedoch Cresent,
        Glasgow C3
    Out-patients Clinic, Baillieston Health Institute,
        Buchanan Street, Baillieston, Glasgow

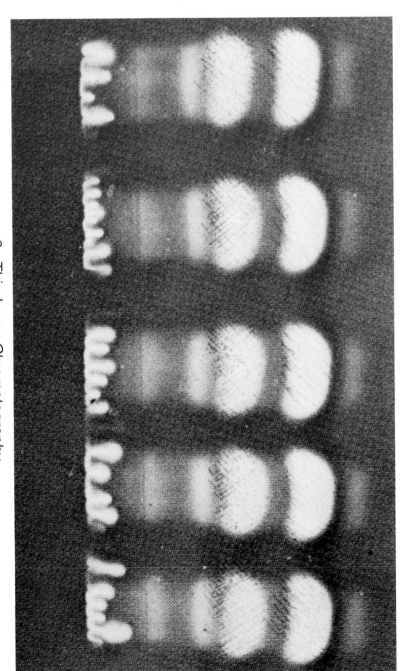

9. Thin Layer Chromatography

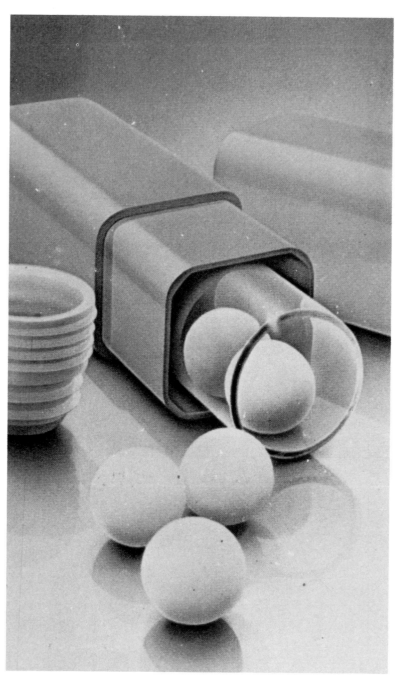

10. Pilules

Liverpool Clinic, The Mossley Hill Hospital,
    Park Avenue, Liverpool L18 8BU

The Bristol Homœopathic Hospital,
    Cotham Road, Cotham, Bristol, BS6 6JU

Tunbridge Wells Homœopathic Hospital,
    Church Road, Tunbridge Wells, Kent

HUGHES, Dr. Richard

Brilliant homœopathic physician, who practised in Brighton and
at the Royal London Homœopathic Hospital and dominated
homœopathy in Britain for many years. Whilst accepting
Hahnemann's concepts, he considered the pathological
symptoms and their modalities to be of prime importance. He
advocated the use of low potencies (less than 30 centesimal),
but with the growing influence of Dr. James Tyler Kent (q.v.),
who favoured high potencies (1M, 10M, CM) a serious rift
developed in the profession.

Dr. Hughes' major work was entitled *Principles and Practise of
Homœopathy* (4 volumes). He died in 1902.

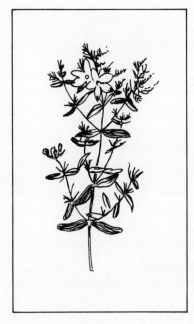

11. Hypericum perforatum

HYPERICUM PERFORATUM

Hypericum. St. John's Wort. Common St. John's Wort.
A member of the Hypericaceæ family, it is an erect, branched
perennial with golden-yellow flowers with minute black spots on
the petals. The plant flourishes in woods, thickets, grassy banks
and gardens. The mother tincture is prepared from the whole
fresh plant.
Used widely in potencies for the treatment of very painful cuts
and wounds, blows to fingers or toes where there is damage to
the nerve tissue, horse-fly bites and bleeding piles. Also used as
a mouth wash, sometimes in combination with Calendula (q.v.).
Symptoms are better when bending the head backwards and
worse indoors, from touch and in the cold and damp.

I

IGNATIA AMARA

Ignatia. St. Ignatius Bean. Strychnos ignatia.
Native plant of the Philippines. The mother tincture is prepared
from the seeds.
Widely used in potencies for the treatment of suppressed grief,
bereavement, depression or shock with weepiness, hysteria or
piercing headache. The particular features are sudden,
spasmodic, erratic pain, generally following some emotional
upset. The patient is disposed to rapid changes in mental
condition and is oversensitive in mind and body. Symptoms are
improved by distribution of heat and are worse in the morning
and with strong odours.

INFINITESIMAL DOSE

Infinitely or very small homœopathic dose in potencies, in
contrast to very large allopathic doses. Hahnemann stated 'the
very smallest doses of medicines chosen for the homœopathic diseases are
each a match for the corresponding disorder. The physician will choose the
homœopathic remedy in just so small a dose as will overcome the disease.'
See Potency; Dilutions.

INSOLUBLE

That which cannot be dissolved in a liquid, especially water
and alcohol. Insoluble materials are homœopathically prepared
by trituration (q.v.).

IPECACUANHA

Ipecac. Ipecacuanha Root.

The mother tincture is prepared from the whole, dried root of the plant. It contains several alkaloids, mainly emetine.

A useful remedy for the treatment of nausea with vomiting, salivation, aversion to food and depression, for example, early morning sickness in pregnancy. Also used for the treatment of spasmodic coughing and nose bleed. Symptoms are worse when lying down.

J

JAHR, Dr. Georg Heinrich

Born in Saxony in 1800, Dr.Jahr qualified at the University of Bonn in 1828. A leading homœopathic physician who practised mainly in Paris over 40 years. He was one of the few German friends of Samuel Hahnemann during his stay in Paris, and he attended him at his death in July 1843. Dr. Jahr wrote many books and papers, including the *Manual of Homœopathic Medicine* (1836) and *A New Homœopathic Pharmacopœia* (1850).

K

KALIUM BICHROMICUM

Kali Bich. Potassium Bichromate. Potassium Dichromate. Bichromate of Potash.

Bright orange-red crystalline salt, prepared from chromium iron ore. Formula: $K_2 Cr_2 O_7$.

A major polycrest remedy for conditions of the nose and throat. Sinus troubles, catarrh with stringy, yellow sputum, dry hard cough, sore throat, nausea and vomiting, particularly after alcohol, measles. Indicated for fat people with fair hair and lacking in energy. Symptoms are worse in hot weather and in the morning.

KALIUM PHOSPHORICUM

Kali Phos. Potassium Phosphate.

White powder. Formula: $K_3 PO_4$. Used in potencies mainly for the treatment of nervous depression, exhaustion or indigestion,

giddiness from exhaustion and weakness during convalescence, bad breath and after influenza. Indicated for shy people with poor memories. Symptoms are worsened by noise and improved by gentle movement and warmth.
See also *Biochemic Remedies*.

KENT, Dr. James Tyler
Born in New York in 1849, Dr. Kent became a leading homœopathic physician. An eminent scholar and teacher, he strictly followed Hahnemannian practices and teachings. He advocated the prescribing of single remedies in high potency. A prolific writer, his major work was the *Repertory of Homœopathic Materia Medica*, published in 1877. Dr. Kent died in 1916.

KNITBONE
See *Symphytum Officinale*.

KORSAKOV POTENTISATION
The Korsakov method of the preparation of homœopathic potencies involves the use of the **same** glass container for successive dilutions rather than separate containers as in the Hahnemannian method. Thus, for centesimal dilutions the container is emptied and 99 drops of alcohol and water are added to what is assumed to be one drop of the previous potency adhering to the surface of the container. Sometimes this method is used for the preparation of very high potencies, but generally it is discouraged.

L

LACHESIS
Bushmaster Snake. Lachesis muta. Lachesis mutus. Surukuku. The mother tincture of this remedy, originally proved by Dr. Constantine Hering (q.v.), is prepared from the poisonous venom of the snake.
Finds special use in the treatment of throat affections, hot flushes and depression in the menopause and menstrual pains. Symptoms are worse from sleep, touch and tight clothing.

LACTOSE

Sugar. Sugar of milk. Formula: $C_{12}H_{22}O_{11}$.

Pure lactose is used homœopathically to produce placebo (q.v.) tablets, pilules, granules or powders, which are then impregnated with the homœopathic medicament.

See also *Trituration*.

LAW OF SIMILARS

This law is the foundation upon which the truth and success of homœopathy is built and is its fundamental principle. It states that a remedy which creates symptoms and conditions in a healthy person will cure a sick person manifesting similar symptoms. Samuel Hahnemann who enunciated this principle, described it in the Latin phrase 'Similia Similibus Curentur' or 'let likes be treated with likes'.

See *Organon; Homœopathy*.

LEAD

See *Plumbum Metallicum*.

LEDUM

Ledum Palustre. Wild Rosemary. Marsh tea.

Member of the Ericaceæ family. A densely branched evergreen shrub with a strong aromatic odour, which thrives in boggy ground. The mother tincture is prepared from the whole fresh plant. Hahnemann described this remedy as suitable for the most part only in chronic conditions in which there is a predominance of coldness.

A remedy frequently used for respiratory and rheumatic conditions, puncture wounds (for example, insect bites, injections or needle injury). Indications are redness, mottling, swelling and throbbing pain. Symptoms are generally worse from heat. Of special benefit to robust people with redness of face who are apt to become discontented.

LIGA MEDICORUM HOMŒOPATHICA INTERNATIONALIS

The International Homœopathic Medical League. The Liga was founded in Holland in 1925 by doctors from different countries. Its purpose is the promotion of the development of homœopathic medicine worldwide and to provide a link between qualified medical practitioners, and also between organisations and people who are interested in·homœopathy. The Liga hold an International Congress at least once in every three years.

LOCUM
    A practitioner (homœopathic doctor, pharmacist or veterinary
    surgeon), who temporarily takes the place of another.

LOT NUMBER
    See *Batch Number*.

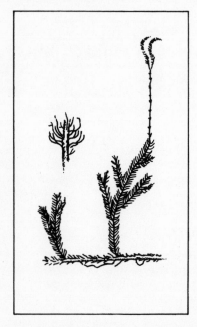

12. Lycopodium clavatum

LYCOPODIUM CLAVATUM
    Lycopodium. Club Moss. Lamb's Tail. Fox Tail.
    A plant with long straggling stems thickly coated with
    hair-pointed leaves, growing abundantly on heathland and
    mountain pastures. One of Samuel Hahnemann's original
    homœopathic remedies. The mother tincture is prepared from
    the crushed spores of the plant.
    A powerful, deep acting remedy, favoured by Hahnemann for
    the treatment of chronic dyspepsia, with strong influence on
    emotional conditions of apprehension and anticipatory anxiety
    for example, pre-examination or interview nerves and stage
    fright. Also used for the treatment of constipation, excessive
    hunger but easily satisfied, flatulence and waterbrash.
    Symptoms are usually worse from 4pm to 8pm. Lycopodium
    subjects tend to have a sallow complexion often with flushed

cheeks and freckles. They are chilly people who hate the cold, with a liking for sweet foods.

M

MANUFACTURER'S LICENCE
Under the provisions of the Medicines Act 1968 and 1971 homœopathic medicines may only be manufactured on premises for which a Manufacturing Licence has been granted by the Department of Health and Social Security. These licences are only granted if the premises conform with certain stringent standards in relation to buildings, equipment and facilities, staffing and expertise and manufacturing and quality control procedures.
See *Product Licence*.

MARIGOLD
See *Calendula Officinalis*.

MATERIA MEDICA
Pharmacopœia. Alphabetical list of homœopathic remedies with their sources, associated symptoms and uses. A collection of homœopathic drug pictures
See *Drug Pictures*; *Repertory*.

MATERIA MEDICA PURA
Title of major work by Dr. Samuel Hahnemann, originally published in two volumes in Leipzig in 1817.

MEDICINE
A substance which is capable of modifying biological activity. Recognising the existence of the body's natural defence mechanism, Hahnemann defined a medicine as a substance which restored the patient to health quicker than when left untreated.

MENTALS
Mental symptoms, which are of special significance to the homœopathic remedy; for example, shyness, tearfulness.
See *Generals*; *Particulars*.

MERCURIUS SOLUBILIS

Merc Sol. Quicksilver. Mercury. Soluble mercury
(Hahnemann). Silver – white, heavy, mobile liquid. Symbol:
Hg. Pure metal produced by roasting mercuric sulphide
(cinnabar ore). Homœopathic remedy proved by Samuel
Hahnemann.

Used in potencies for many conditions, including bad breath,
body odour with abnormal sweating, sore throat, diarrhœa,
abscesses, chicken pox, mumps and genito-urinary treatment.
Symptoms are often worse at night and at extreme temperatures
and improved by dry moderate heat.

MIASM

A term introduced by Hahnemann for a condition which may
be inherited or acquired. Postulated as the manifestation of all
chronic diseases. Miasm cannot be properly defined in modern
medical terms.

MICROCRYSTALLOGRAPHY

A method by which mother tinctures may be studied or
identified, based on their crystallisation as mixtures with
chromium or nickel salt solutions. The crystal patterns
produced are varied, complex, highly organised and exhibit a
perfect, natural beauty.
See *Chromatography*.

MODALITIES

Aggravations (q.v.) or modifying influences (ameliorations)
which influence the choice of a homœopathic remedy.
Aggravations are denoted: >; ameliorations: <.
See *Physical Modalities*; *Thermal Modalities*; *Time Modalities*.

MOTHER TINCTURES

Liquids prepared by the maceration, ageing, compression and
filtration of selected animal, vegetable and sometimes biological
materials, or the solution of soluble minerals in alcohol and
water mixtures. Mother tinctures are clear liquids ranging in
colour from pale straw to dark brown or dark red. Mother
tinctures, denoted by the Greek letter Ø may be described as the
homœopathic medicament in its most concentrated form. They
are the starting material in the preparation of homœopathic
potencies (q.v.). Some mother tinctures are used in undiluted
form in homœopathic treatment (sometimes called phytotherapy)
and others are incorporated in oitments or creams.

N

NATRUM MURIATICUM

Nat. Mur. Sodium Chloride. Common Salt. Formula: Na Cl.
Prepared in pure form as white crystals, granules or powder
from naturally occurring rock salt, from the evaporation of brine
from underground salt deposits or from sea water.
A major polycrest (q.v.) remedy associated with exhaustion and
craving for excessive salt in the diet. In potencies it is
prescribed mainly for sinus troubles, sneezy colds, runny nose,
cold sores, exhaustion and herpes of the mouth.

NOSODES

A class of homœopathic medicines prepared from morbid or
diseased tissues, for example, pus, which are usually included in
the various Materia Medica. The bowel nosodes are a special
type of nosode (q.v.).
Nosodes are potentised in the normal way and do not contain
the 'live' or active organisms and therefore they are quite safe.
They are rarely prescribed in the acute stages of a disease, but
usually prophylactically and where a patient claims to have
'*never been well since*' suffering from a particular disease. Nosodes
demonstrate the analogy between homœopathy and
immunology. They are usually prescribed in a single dose in the
30th potency or higher.
Nosodes can be distinguished from other homœopathic
medicines in that their names all end with the suffix –inum, for
example Influenzinum; Medorrhinum.
See *Bowel Nosodes*.

NOSODES, BOWEL

Special category of nosodes originally developed by Dr. Edward
Bach (q.v.) and Dr. John Paterson, a Glasgow physician and
bacteriologist. Remedies derived from cultures of stools which
contain bacteria from the intestines.
See *Nosodes*.

NUTRIENT

A nourishing substance or food.

NUX VOMICA

Nux Vom. Poison Nut. Strychnos Nux Vomica. Colubrina.
A tree with a crooked trunk which grows in the East Indes and
Northern Australia. The fruit is an orange berry containing five

seeds and it is these seeds which, after drying, are used to prepare the mother tincture. They contain several alkaloids, but mainly strychnine which is very poisonous giving seizure and convulsions.

A most important polycrest remedy especially, though not exclusively, for men (particularly the overworked executive). Used mainly for the treatment of nervous indigestion, morning liverishness or hangover, constipation, itching piles, stomach pain, feeling of weight on the stomach and shooting pains. The patient is characterised as slim, pale, dark haired, over anxious and quarrelsome, who moves briskly and talks rapidly. Symptoms are worse in the cold and early mornings, after intellectual effort and after meals, and better in the evening with warmth and with sleep.

O

ONION
See *Allium cepa*.

ORGANON
Samuel Hahnemann's greatest written work, entitled *Organon of Rational Healing* (later the title was changed to *Organon of the Healing Art*), published in Dresden in 1810. The book, which ran to six editions, contained a complete exposition of his new homœopathic therapy and laid down the Law of Similars, which is the essential principle.
See *Law of Similars*.

P

PALLIATIVE
A remedy which alleviates or suppresses the symptoms of a disease without curing the disease.

PARACELSUS, Dr. Theophastus (1493–1541)
Dr. Theophastus von Hohenheim Bombast, who adopted the pseudonym Paracelsus. Swiss physician and philosopher who was for some time lecturer in medicine in Basle. In many

respects his life resembled that of Samuel Hahnemann in that he was a brilliant physician, a leading medical reformer of his day, he led a wandering life and wrote many medical books and pamphlets. His writings foreshadowed the principles of homœopathy and modern pharmacology in a simple way and he is sometimes regarded as the patron of holistic (q.v.) medicine.

PARTICULARS

Particular or 'local' symptoms; for example, pain in the stomach, or headache, affecting specific parts or individual organs of the body. See *Generals*; *Mentals*.

PATHOLOGY

The study of disease.

PHARMACEUTICAL FORMS

Preparations of medicines in forms suitable for administration to the patient. These forms include tablets, pilules, granules, suppositories and liquids.

PHARMACOPŒIA

Homœopathic medicines are prepared in accordance with the methods described in the British or American editions of the Homœopathic Pharmacopœia.
See *Materia Medica*.

PHOSPHORUS

Red Phosphorus. Symbol: P.
Allotropic form of the element. Red to violet powder. Extracted from naturally occurring phosphate rock.
Indicated in tall pale, fair haired people. Used in potencies mainly for the treatment of dry cough, bronchitis and hypersensitivity.

PHYSICAL MODALITIES

Reactions of patient to touch, movement, rest, exertion, etc.
See *Modalities*.

For example: Touch

Better for:		*Worse for:*
Bryonia	(pressure)	Apis Mel
Calc. Carb.	—	Arnica
Chelidonium	—	Cantharis
	(pressure)	China

Better for:		*Worse for*:
China	(pressure)	Ferrum Phos.
Colocynth	(pressure)	Hepar Sulph.

PHYTOLACCA DECANDRA

Phytolacca. Phytolacca americana. Virginian Poke. Pigeon berry. American nightshade.

Member of the Phytolaccaceæ or Pokeweed family. A tall, herbaceous perennial with a thick, ribbed stem and large oval leaves. Greenish or pink flowers with fruit consisting of clusters of purplish-black berries. A native plant of North America. The mother tincture is prepared from the entire plant, including the berries.

A useful remedy in the treatment of sore throat, mastitis, inability to swallow, loss of voice in singers and speakers, shooting burning pains likened to electric shocks, after effects of rheumatism and constipation in the aged.

Symptoms are worse from damp or exposure to night air, swallowing and hot drinks. Most likely to benefit those people who shrink from mental exertion or who are indifferent to life.

PILULE

Pilule. Pill. A traditional pharmaceutical form of homœopathic medicines in the shape of a small sphere, 4 millimetres in diameter and 3-5 milligrammes in weight, suitable for administration to the patient. Now availabe in the highest standard of purity, pilules are favoured by many homœopaths.

PLACEBO

A non-active, unmedicated material used to satisfy a patient or as a control in clinical trials (q.v.) designed to test the efficacy of a particular treatment.

See *Lactose*.

PLACEBO EFFECT

A psychologically induced cure.

PLASTIC

See *Containers*.

PLUMBUM METALLICUM

Plumbum met. Lead metal. Symbol: Pb.

Bluish-white, silvery grey metal, extracted mainly from the mineral galena (lead sulphide). Prepared by trituration of the pure powdered metal.

This remedy is mainly for muscle spasms or muscle weakness.

POISON NUT
See *Nux Vomica*.

POLYCREST
Frequently used remedies with symptoms related to many different systems. Examples are: Ignatia, Natrum Muriaticum, Nux Vomica, Phosphorus, Pulsatilla and Sepia and Sulphur.

POSOLOGY
Study of the quantities or dosages in which homœopathic medicines are administered. See *Dosage*.

POTASSIUM
See *Kalium compounds*.

POISON IVY
See *Rhus toxicodendron*.

POTENCIES
Samuel Hahnemann determined by systematic experimentation that by progressively reducing the quantity of drug administered, he could make the treatment safe and minimise the aggravations (q.v.), yet retain its therapeutic activity. The drug appeared to be stronger – or more potent – as a result of dilution, and therefore, he named these dilutions 'potencies'. Generally, the low potencies are short-acting, whereas the high potencies are longer-acting over a wider and deeper range of symptoms, particularly chronic (q.v.) conditions.

The most common potencies employed are:

Low Potencies
3x 6x 12x 30x 3c 6c
Medium (or transitional) Potencies
(6c) 12c 30c 200c
High Potencies
(200c) 1,000c (or 1M) 10M 50M CM

POTENTISATION
The procedure by which substances are transformed into potencies (q.v.) suitable for use in homœopathic treatment.

Manufacturers of homœopathic medicines carry out this vital operation under specially controlled conditions to ensure the integrity of their products.

See *Potency*; *Quality Control*.

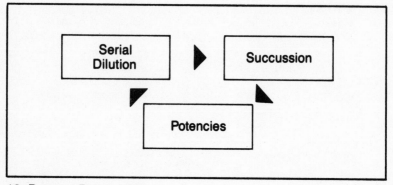

13. Potency Preparation

POTENCY

Potencies are a fundamentally important feature of all homœopathic remedies and their prescribing. The potentisation process by which they are prepared involves the serial or sequential dilution of the mother tincture prepared from the original substance or source (q.v.) with a mixture of pure alcohol and water. Each dilution is followed by succussion (q.v.), that is, vigorous shaking with impact.

There are two methods of dilution – decimal and centesimal. The decimal series of potencies are governed by successive dilutions of one part of mother tincture to ten parts of alcohol/water; these are denoted x (or D) potencies. The centesimal series of potencies are governed by successive dilutions of one part of mother tincture to one hundred parts alcohol/water; these are denoted c (or cH) potencies.

Substances which are insoluble in alcohol/water mixtures are potentised in their solid form with pure lactose powder by the process of trituration (q.v.).

It must be remembered that potency cannot be defined in terms of dilution alone, since potency numbers refer to the number of succussions. For example, potencies of 6(c) and 12x have the same dilution, but the former involves 6 succussions and the latter, 12 succussions.

See *Dilution* of Homœopathic Potencies. *Trituration. Succussion. Symbols. Attenuation.*

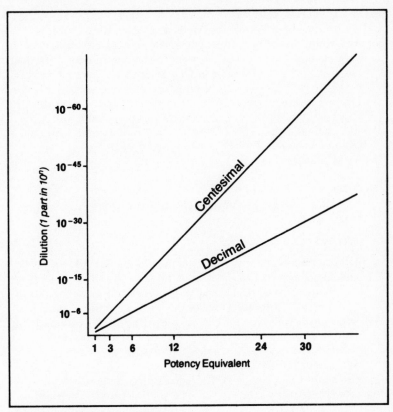

14. Potency Equivalents/Dilution

PRE–POTENCIES
Potencies of one potency number lower than the prime potencies (for example: 5,29) prepared for stock purposes.

PRECIPITATE
Solid particles which separate from a clear solution. Some mother tinctures (q.v.) produce a precipitate which may appear as a cloudiness of the clear solution on storage. The precipitate may be separated by filtration.

PRIME POTENCIES
The most commonly prescribed potencies (q.v.), which are generally considered to correspond with peak levels of therapeutic efficacy.
See *Potencies*.

PRODUCT LICENCE

Under the provisions of the Medicines Act 1968 & 1971, all medicines, including homœopathic medicines, may only be manufactured, advertised, sold and distributed under a Product Licence issued by the Department of Health. Those medicines available before 1968 were granted Product Licences of Right. Product Licences are granted for medicines which meet the standards laid down in respect of safety, purity and effectiveness. A product licence number may be recognised on a label by two sets of four digits separated by an oblique stroke. See *Manufacturers Licence.*

PROVER

A healthy person who participates in the proving (q.v.) of a homœopathic medicine.

PROVING

A procedure to test a potential homœopathic remedy on healthy persons. The object of this trial is to catalogue all symptoms and characteristics which can be genuinely associated with the substance. Hahnemann, his family and his followers, bravely pioneered this field at great risk to their health to *prove* many of the well known remedies of homœopathy in a systematic manner. The original homœopathic remedy proved by Hahnemann was Cinchona (q.v.).

The result of a proving is a 'drug picture' (q.v.) which is listed with others to make up a Materia Medica (q.v.). The word *proving* is derived from the German verb *prüfen* – to test.

PSORA

Latent predisposition to a disease.

PULSATILLA NIGRICANS

Pulsatilla. Wind Flower. Meadow anemone. Pasque flower. Member of the Ranunculaceæ (Buttercup) family, it is considered by botanists to be most primitive. The mother tincture is prepared from the whole, fresh flowering plant in the spring or autumn.

This most effective polycrest remedy is particularly favoured with women, particularly gentle, weepy blondes, although not exclusively. 'Pulsatilla types' may be mild people becoming irritable.

Worse in a warm room, better for moving about slowly, with periodic sick headaches and chronic catarrh. Used mainly for the treatment of weepiness, particularly in children, menstrual problems, change of life, shingles, hayfever, headaches (especially overnight) and styes. Symptoms are improved in open air and expression of sympathy. The Pulsatilla child or girl may be sweet, charming and rather emotional who feels worse in the evening. It is sometimes called the *sunset remedy*.

Q

QUALITY CONTROL
Stringent controls and laboratory tests carried out at every stage of manufacture of homœopathic medicines, from raw materials to finished product, to ensure a high standard of purity.
Techniques such as thin layer chromotography are employed to check the identity of mother tinctures. Hahnemann stated, '*the physician can only be sure about the healing properties of a medicine when it is made as pure and as perfect as possible.*'
See *Manufacturer's Licence*; *Chromatography*.

QUIN, Dr. Frederick Harvey Foster (1799–1878).
Qualified in medicine at the University of Edinburgh, after attending school in Putney. Travelled extensively in Europe and was appointed physician to Prince Leopold of Saxe-Coburg (later King of Belgium). Became a disciple of Hahnemann and introduced homœopathy into Great Britain in the late 1820s. He wrote extensively and established the British Homœopathic Society (later Faculty of Homœopathy) in 1844. Founded the London Homœopathic Hospital (later Royal) at 32 Golden Square in 1849.

R

REMEDY PICTURE
See *Drug Picture*.

REPERTORY
An index of drug symptoms recorded in homœopathic Materia Medica, each heading listing those drugs known to cause the symptoms. Prominent symptoms are often printed in **heavy** or **black type** to distinguish them.

REMEDY

A substance used in the treatment of disease. See list of 50 commonly used homœopathic remedies, page 65.

RHUS TOXICODENDRON

Rhus Tox. Poison Ivy. Poison Oak. Rhus radicans.
Member of the Sumac family. Very poisonous shrub or vine indigenous to the east coast of America. The mother tincture is prepared from its leaves, which are dark green, freshly gathered just before flowering and just after sunset.
One of the most effective and widely used homœopathic remedies, its potencies are used for the treatment of rheumatism, sprains of the joints and tendons, lumbago, sciatica, herpes of the lips, shingles, chicken pox and mumps. Patients may be restless, depressed, apprehensive at night and have a preference for solitude. All symptoms are worse for fatigue, lack of movement, cold and damp and improved by hot, dry weather.

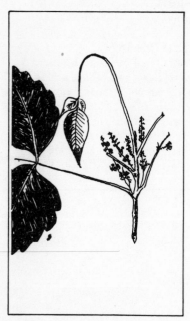

15. Rhus toxicodendron

RUTA GRAVEOLENS

Ruta Grav. Rue. Bitterwort. Herb of Grace. Herbygrass. Common Rue.
Medicinal herb known to early civilisations. Strong smelling

usually glaucous, woody based, shrub-like perennial with yellow
flowers having widely-spaced petals. Found throughout Europe
in hilly country, rocks and old walls.

Homœopathic potencies are indicated for eye strain and fatigue
with blurred vision, burning fractures, dislocations, bruised
bones, aching and tightness in the chest and eyestrain followed
by headache. All symptoms are worse for cold, damp conditions
and on initial movement after resting. Most beneficial for those
with anxiety and dissatisfied with self and others.

ROYAL PATRONAGE
Homœopathy has received the valued support of the Royal
Family for six generations, since Dr. Stapf, a colleague of
Samuel Hahnemann, travelled to England to treat Queen
Adelaide (consort to King William IV) in 1835.

Its principal patrons include Prince Albert (Consort to Queen
Victoria), Queen Mary (Consort to George V), King George VI
and H.M. The Queen Mother, H.M. The Queen, HRH Prince
Charles and HRH Princess Margaret.

S

SAFETY OF HOMŒOPATHIC MEDICINES
See *Side Effects. Toxicity.*

SAMUEL HAHNEMANN
See *Hahnemann.*

SARCODES
Homœopathic attenuations of wholesome organs or tissues
obtained from healthy animals.

SEQUENTIAL DILUTION
See *Potency.*

SHELF LIFE
See *Stability. Storage.*

SIDE EFFECTS
There are no dangerous or unwanted side effects caused by
homœopathic medicines. They are safe and non-addictive, even
for babies and young children. Although the medicines are quite

safe, Department of Health regulations require a warning stated on the label of *all* medicines, including homœopathic medicines.

SILICEA
Silica. Pure Flint. Silicon Dioxide. Silicic Anhydride. Formula: SiO_2. White powder or transparent crystals. Occurs naturally as agate, flint, quartz, sand, and tridymite.
A polycrest remedy prepared by trituration, used mainly for the treatment of boils and abscesses, chronic headaches, sinus troubles and body odour. Most beneficial to people with fine skin and pale complexion who find mental effort difficult. Symptoms are worse from heat and in the evening and better in the open air or from cold applications.

SIMILARS
See *Law of Similars*.

SIMILLIMUM
The correct homœopathic medicine which matches the overall symptom picture of the patient.

SOLUBLE
That which can be dissolved in a liquid, especially water or alcohol or mixtures. Solubility is usually expressed as a number of grammes of the substance which will dissolve in one litre of the liquid at a given temperature.

SOURCES OF HOMŒOPATHIC MEDICINES
Most homœopathic medicines are derived from natural sources of plant, mineral or animal origin. Plants are collected from their natural habitats or grown 'organically' in nurseries without the use of pesticides or artificial fertilisers. The whole plant or its flowers, leaves, berries, fruits, seeds, bark or roots may be used in the preparation of the remedies. Minerals are mainly naturally occurring elements, mineral salts or ores. Examples (q.v.) of each raw material source are as follows:

Plant : Arnica; Belladonna; Gelsemium; Hypericum; Euphrasia; Calendula; Symphytum (q.v.).
Mineral: Calcium Carbonate; Cuprum metallicum; Kali phosphoricum; Sulphur; Natrum muriaticum (q.v.); Nitric acid.
Animal : Apis mellifica; Lachesis; Sepia (q.v.).
See *A-Z List of Homœopathic Medicines. Nosodes.*

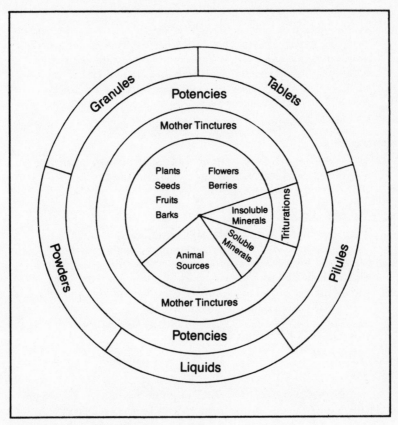

16. Sources of homœopathic medicines

STABILITY

Most homœopathic medicines, if properly stored, are very stable and retain their effectiveness for long periods. The nominal *shelf life* of homœopathic medicines, agreed with the Department of Health and Social Security, is five years, but many medicines can be stored for considerably longer periods.
See *Storage*.

STAPF, Dr. Johann

Close friend and pupil of Dr. Samuel Hahnemann. Born in Naumberg in 1788, he corresponded with Hahnemann until his death. Proved over 30 homœopathic medicines. He wrote many dissertations and articles on homœopathy. In 1835 he visited England to treat Queen Adelaide at Windsor.

STORAGE

Homœopathic medicines should be kept away from direct light, in a cool place. They should be kept away from strong smelling substances, such as camphor, perfumes or disinfectants. The container cap should be kept firmly in position; spilled tablets or pilules should be rejected. The medicines should not be handled as contamination could lower their efficacy. See *Stability*.

SUCCUS

Juice. A liquid derived from animal tissue or from plants, sometimes produced as an intermediate in the preparation of mother tinctures (q.v.).

SUCCUSSION

Violent shaking with impact carried out at each stage of sequential dilution in the preparation of a homœopathic potency. Originally, the impact was provided by striking the vial against a leather bound book, but nowadays mechanical means are employed. The impact energises the dilution and is a vital part of the potentisation (q.v.) procedure.

SUGAR OF MILK.

See *Lactose*.

SULPHUR

Sublimated sulphur. Flowers of sulphur. Symbol: S. Fine yellow crystalline powder. Known since early times. The element occurs in the free state in nature. One of Samuel Hahnemann's original homœopathic remedies, it is associated with chronic disease. Used extensively for the treatment of certain skin troubles such as itching skin, eczema, boils, burning and itching piles and inflamed orifices, chronic catarrh and constipation. Symptoms are worse for rest, washing, and standing and better for warm, dry weather.

SUSS – HAHNEMANN, Dr. Leopold

Only son of Samuel Hahnemann's daughter, Amalie. Dr. Leopold Suss-Hahnemann adopted his surname in deference to his grandfather after his parents divorced. He practised homœopathic medicine in London until he retired to Ventnor, Isle of Wight, where he died in 1914. His direct descendants now live in Crowborough, Sussex.

SYMBOLS (HOMŒOPATHIC)
Ø	Mother Tincture
<	amelioration
>	aggravation
X(x)	decimal potency
c	centesimal potency
c.H	centesimal Hahnemann
K	Korsakov

SYMPHYTUM OFFICINALE
Symphytum. Comfrey. 'Knitbone'.
Member of the Boraginaceæ family. A leafy perennial plant, branched from its base, with clusters of yellow/white, pink or purple flowers. Grows in damp meadows and marshes in most parts of Europe.
An old homœopathic remedy used to assist the healing of bone fractures and injuries, for the treatment of deep-seated pains in the bones and rheumatic and arthritic conditions resulting from bone fractures.

SYMPTOMS
Discernible changes in body functions of the patient indicating disease. The homœopath regards the symptoms of a disease as a manifestation of the body's fight against that disease, that is the natural curative process. Homœopathic treatment seeks, therefore, to stimulate those symptoms, rather than to suppress them. The homœopathic physician classifies symptoms into 'Generals' (q.v.), Particulàrs (q.v.), and Mentals (q.v.). He will also note the rare and peculiar features of symptoms and take the totality of symptoms into consideration to prescribe the correct remedy.
See *Modalities*; *Proving*.

T

TABLETS
Common pharmaceutical form for the administration of homœopathic medicines. Produced by the compression of a mixture of pure lactose and sucrose, as white double convex tablets, each weighing 0.1 grammes.
Note. Medicated tablets should not be handled with bare hands to avoid contamination.
See *Pilules*.

THIN LAYER CHROMATOGRAPHY
See *Chromatography*.

THERAPEUTIC
Having curative properties. Therapeutics is the branch of medicine concerned with the application of remedies in the treatment of disease, including dosage and administration.

THERMAL MODALITIES
Reactions of patient to heat and cold. See *Modalities*.

Examples:

Cold	**Warmth or Heat**
Better for:	*Better for*:
Antim Tart.	Arsen Alb.
Baptisia	Aurum Met.
Bryonia	Belladonna
Carbo Veg.	Calc. Carb.
Gelsemium	Calc. Phos.
Lachesis	Causticum
Natrum Mur.	China
Pulsatilla	Drosera
	Ferrum Phos.
Worse for:	Kali Bich.
Arnica	Lycopodium
Hepar Sulph.	Nux Vomica
Hypericum	Phos. Acid
Ruta	Phytolacca
Spongia	Rhus Tox.
	Sepia
	Silicea
	Sulphur
	Veratrum Alb.
	Worse for:
	Antim. Crud.
	Apis mel.
	Chamomilla
	Drosera (cough).

THUJA OCCIDENTALIS
Thuja. Arbor Vitæ. Tree of Life.
Slow growing shrub or conifer. The mother tincture is prepared from the fresh, green branches.

An important homœopathic remedy for chronic disease,
introduced by Samuel Hahnemann.
The Thuja patient is dark skinned and dark haired with a
strong, obstinate personality. Main uses are for the treatment of
warts, body odour, morning headaches with aversion to food
and pain with the frequent passing of water. Symptoms are
worse in the early morning or mid-afternoon and from cold and
better when drawing up a limb.

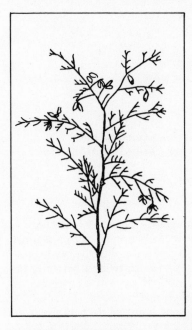

17. Thuja occidentalis

TIME MODALITIES for symptoms at the peak of their activity

About midnight	– Rhus tox.
Midnight to 3 am	– Drosera
1 am to 2 am	– Arsen Alb.
Before 3 am	– Nux Vomica, Thuja
2 am to 3 am	– Kali Bich.
About 3 am	– Bryonia
3 am to 4 am	– Hypericum
10 am to 11 am	– Gelsemium, Natrum Mur.
About 11 am	– Ipecacuanha, Sulphur
Morning	– Ignatia
About 2 pm	– Calc. Carb.
About 3 pm	– Belladonna
About 4 pm	– Pulsatilla (fever)

4 pm to 5 pm	– Carbo Veg.
4 pm to 6 pm	– Apis Mel.
5 pm to 6 pm	– Hepar Sulph., Phosphorus (fever)
About 7 pm	– Rhus tox.
About 9 pm	– Bryonia (fever)
10 pm to midnight	– Belladonna
Before midnight	– Aconite, Carbo Veg., Graphites, Pulsatilla

TINCTURES
See *Mother Tinctures*.

TOTALITY OF SYMPTOMS
The sum total of the sensations and observable changes in the organism.

TOXIC
Poisonous. Many of the sources of homœopathic medicines are toxic in their raw state, although the finished medicines are always non-toxic and quite safe.
See *Side Effects*.

TRITURATION
A process to produce homœopathic medicines from insoluble substances. The active ingredient is finely ground with a neutral substance (usually lactose) using a mortar and pestle, to yield a powder which can be formed into tablets or pilules. Mixtures of one part of the active ingredient with ten parts of the neutral substance are used to produce the decimal series of potencies (q.v.) and mixtures of one part to one hundred parts of the active ingredient for the centesimal series of potencies (q.v.).

TYLER, Dr. Margaret
Leading practitioner of homœopathy for more than forty years at the Royal London Homœopathic Hospital, until her death in 1943. Her book *Drug Pictures of Homœopathic Remedies* is still a valuable source of information.

TYPES
See *Constitutional Remedy*.

U

UNIT DOSE
See *Dosage*.

URTICA URENS
Stinging Nettle. Small nettle.
Member of the Urticaceæ family. Grows profusely in gardens,
waste ground and roadsides throughout Europe. A leafy annual
with stinging hairs. Mother tincture is prepared from the fresh,
flowering plant.
Used mainly for the treatment of urticaria, itchy skin, blotches,
sunburn, stinging burns and scalds and insect bites. Urtica has
also been used for gout and affections of the spleen. Symptoms
are worsened by cold, contact with water and at night.

V

VALERIANA OFFICINALIS
Valerian.
A robust perennial herb with an erect, grooved stem about 1m
(3-4 ft) high. Member of the Valerianacea family. Dense,
branched clusters of numerous, small white or pale pink flowers,
blooming in May, June and July. Grows in meadows and woods
throughout Europe, Asia and Ireland. On drying it has a strong
turpentine-like smell. Its roots are used to prepare the mother
tincture, the principal constituents of which are glucosides and
valerianic acid.
A useful homœopathic remedy for the treatment of headaches
resulting from nervous tension, as a tranquillising agent and
nerve tonic. Good secondary remedy for despair and pessimism,
accompanied by restlessness. Symptoms are worse at night and
early morning and better in the afternoon.

VITAL FORCE
The term used by Samuel Hahnemann (q.v.) to describe the
inherited natural curative powers within the human body.
Homœopathic medicines seek to stimulate this force or energy
to overcome the disease. Hahnemann stated '*it is certain that the
vital forces may achieve victory over disease without inflicting losses on the
body, provided they are assisted and directed in their action by a properly
selected homœopathic remedy.*'

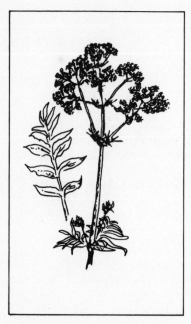

18. Valeriana officinalis

VEGETABLE CHARCOAL
See *Carbo Vegetabilis.*

VERATRUM ALBUM
Veratrum alb. White Hellebore. White False Helleborine.
An erect perennial with a cluster of many whitish or
greenish-yellow flowers, flowering from June to August. Grows
in hills, mountains and fields in most parts of Europe.
A major remedy known to the ancient Greeks, it was the subject
of Samuel Hahnemann's thesis delivered at the University of
Leipzig in 1811 to secure his professorial post. Indicated for
mental illness, all kinds of neuralgia, collapse or shock with
extreme chill and pallor, and severe menstrual tension. Most
likely to benefit are those suffering from fright, shock or injury
with restlessness or resentment.

VETERINARY HOMŒOPATHY
The application of homœopathy in the treatment of sick
animals. Veterinary homœopathy requires not only a careful
study of the animal's symptoms, but an acute observation by
the owner of its behaviour and temperament. Homœopathic
treatment is equally effective for all types of animals, including
pedigree cattle, thoroughbred racehorses and household pets.

60

Veterinary homœopathy has been more widely practised in recent years and the growing interest is demonstrated by the formation of the British Association of Homœopathic Veterinary Surgeons.

W

WEIR, Sir John (1879–1971)
Eminent homœopathic physician, who was appointed physician to H.M. King George V and Queen Mary in 1918. Born in 1879, Dr. Weir qualified in Glasgow in 1906 and subsequently studied in the U.S.A. From 1910 until his retirement he was a consultant physician at the Royal London Homœopathic Hospital and he became President of the Faculty of Homœopathy in 1923. He died in 1971.

WHOLISTIC MEDICINE
Holistic medicine. A general term used to describe all alternative or complementary medicines or therapies which are

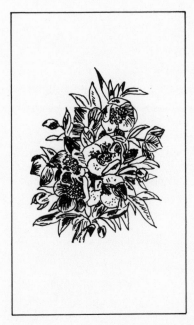

19. Veratrum album

concerned with all aspects of a patient and his or her life rather than a particular illness. Hence, the *whole person*.

X

X POTENCIES
Decimal series of homœopathic potencies derived from dilutions or attenuations of mother tinctures in the ratio of 1:10.
See *Potencies*; *Dilutions*.

X-RAYS
Sometimes used in potencies of ethyl alcohol which has been exposed to x-rays for a variety or conditions.

Y

YELLOW JASMINE
See *Gelsemium sempervirens*.

Z

ZINCUM METALLICUM
Zinc. Symbol: Zn.
Bluish–white, lustrous metal known since very early times. Potencies are prepared by trituration (q.v.). Occurs naturally in calamine or zinc blende.
One of Hahnemann's original homœopathic remedies associated with chronic conditions. Remedy for agitation, convulsions with great depression between fits, paralysis and meningitis. The patient is oversensitive to the least noise and is worse for touch or after food.

Abbreviations

a.c.	before food
Ag	silver
A.I.H.	American Institute of Homœopathy
aq.	aqua (water)
ante	before
Au	gold (aurum)
B.A.H.P.	British Association of Homœopathic Pharmacists
B.A.H.V.S.	British Association of Homœopathic Veterinary Surgeons
B.H.A.	British Homœopathic Association
b.i.d.	twice a day
C	carbon (graphites)
c (or C)	Centesimal potency (Great Britain)
Ca	calcium
cH (or CH)	Centesimal potency Hahnemann (Continent of Europe)
cf.	Compare with
Cu	copper (cuprum)
D	Decimal potency (Continent of Europe)
d.d.	daily
Fe	iron (ferrum)
F.F. Hom	Fellow of the Faculty of Homœopathy
F.R.C.P.	Fellow of the Royal College of Physicians
G.H.H.	Glasgow Homœopathic Hospital
G.P.	General practitioner
H.D.F.	Homœopathic Development Foundation
Hg	mercury
Hom.	Homœopathy
K	potassium (kali)
K	Korsakov
mg	milligramme
ml	millilitre

M.B.	Bachelor of Medicine
M.D.	Doctor of Medicine
m.d.u.	to be used as directed
M.F.Hom	Member of the Faculty of Homœopathy
mist.	a mixture
M.P.S.	Member of the Pharmaceutical Society
M.R.C.V.S.	Member of the Royal College of Veterinary Surgeons
Na	sodium (natrum)
n. et m.	night and morning
N.H.S.	National Health Service
ol.	oil
P	phosphorus
Pb	lead (plumbum)
p.c.	after food
Ph.D.	Doctor of Philosophy
p.r.n.	when required
q.d.s.	four times a day
q.v.	which see
R.L.H.H.	Royal London Homœopathic Hospital
S	sulphur
succ.	succus; juice
T.H.S.	The Hahnemann Society
t.d.s.	three times a day
T.L.C.	Thin layer chromatography
tinct.	a tincture
T.M.	Mother Tincture (also Ø)
ung.	ointment
x (or X)	Decimal potency
Zn	zinc (zincum)

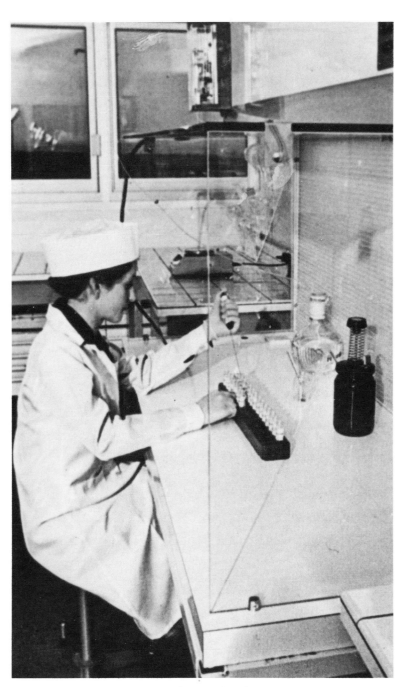

20. Potentisation

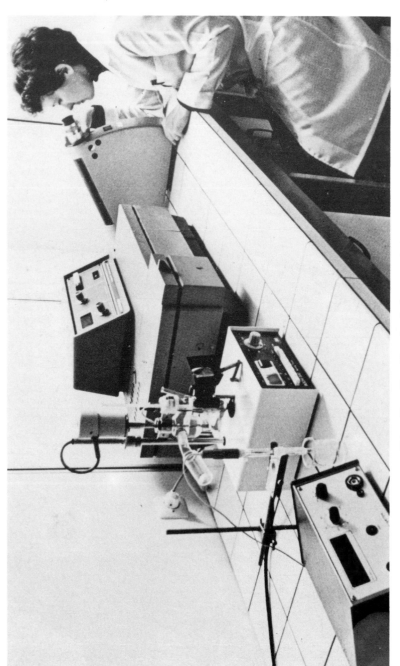

21. Quality Control Apparatus

Fifty Most Commonly Used Homœopathic Medicines

Abbreviation	Full Name	Common Name	Common Uses
1. Aconite	Aconitum napellus	Monkshood	Effects of fear and fright; sore throat; chicken pox; neuralgia.
2. Actæa rac	Actæa racemosa	Baneberry	Neuralgia; stiff neck; effects of over exertion; change of life.
3. Allium cepa	Allium cepa	Onion	Common colds with sneezing and watering eyes.
4. Apis mel.	Apis mellifica	Honey bee	Insect stings; swollen ankles; burning pains.
5. Argent Nit.	Argentum Nitricum	Silver Nitrate	Dyspepsia; acidity; mental strain; headache; chronic laryngitis.
6. Arnica	Arnica montana	Leopard's Bane	Bruises; shock; before surgery or dental treatment; exhaustion.
7. Arsen alb.	Arsenicum album	Arsenious Oxide	Diarrhœa; vomiting; mild food poisoning; hay fever.
8. Belladonna	Atropa belladonna	Deadly Nightshade	Throbbing pains; facial neuralgia; sore throat; measles; mumps.
9. Berberis	Berberis aquifolium/ Berberis vulgaris	Barberry	Anxiety; fear; depression.
10. Bryonia	Bryonia alba	White Bryony	Muscular pain; chesty colds; dry cough.

	Abbreviation	Full Name	Common Name	Common Uses
11.	Calc Carb.	Calcarea Carbonica	Calcium Carbonate	Excessive appetite; profuse periods; acne; cramp.
12.	Calc Fluor.	Calcarea Fluorica	Calcium Fluoride	Cracked joints; thick catarrh; bleeding piles.
13.	Calc Phos.	Calcarea Phosphorica	Calcium Phosphate	Slow healing fractures; severe stomach pains after eating; brain fag.
14.	Calendula	Calendula officinalis	Marigold	Healing cuts and sores.
15.	Cantharis	Cantharis vesicatoria	Spanish fly	Burns and scalds before blisters form, e.g. sunburn; cystitis.
16.	Carbo veg.	Carbo vegetabilis	Vegetable charcoal	Indigestion with flatulence; acne; hoarseness; general debility.
17.	Chamomilla	Chamomilla	Wild chamomile	Teething infants; nausea; migraine.
18.	Cocculus	Cocculus indicus	Cocculus	Travel sickness; nausea; physical and mental strain.
19.	Colchicum	Colchicum autumnale	Autumn crocus	Irritability; gout.
20.	Cuprum met.	Cuprum metallicum	Copper	Cramp; nausea; poor circulation; whooping cough.
21.	Drosera	Drosera rotundifolia	Sundew	Persistent hoarse, barking cough; tickling cough; whooping cough.
22.	Euphrasia	Euphrasia officinalis	Eyebright	Inflamed, watering eyes; conjunctivitis; measles; German measles.
23.	Ferr Phos.	Ferrum Phosphoricum	Iron Phosphate	Nose bleed; hot flushes; varying appetite; fear.

	Abbreviation	Full Name	Common Name	Common Uses
24.	Gelsemium	Gelsemium sempervirens	Yellow Jasmine	Influenza; sore throat; runny nose; measles; examination or interview nerves.
25.	Graphites	Graphites	Black Lead	Cracked, weeping eczema; chapped, unhealthy skin; constipation.
26.	Hamamelis	Hamamelis virginica	Witch Hazel	Chilblains; varicose veins; heavy periods; bleeding piles.
27.	Hepar Sulph.	Hepar Sulphuris	Calcium Sulphide	Wheezing; abscesses; boils; croup; skin sensitive to touch.
28.	Hypericum	Hypericum perforatum	St. John's Wort	Blows to fingers and toes; very painful cuts and wounds; bleeding piles.
29.	Ignatia	Ignatia amara	St. Ignatius Bean	Bereavement; shock; weepiness; hysteria; piercing headaches.
30.	Ipecac	Ipecacuanha	Ipecacuanha	Constant nausea and sickness; morning sickness; nose bleed; spasmodic coughing.
31.	Kali Bich.	Kali bichromicum	Potassium Bichromate	Stringy, yellow sputum; sore throat; dry cough; measles.
32.	Kali Phos.	Kali phosphoricum	Potassium Phosphate	Exhaustion; indigestion; weakness during convalescence and after influenza.
33.	Lachesis	Lachesis muta	Bushmaster Snake Venom	Throat infections; hot flushes; depression during menopause.
34.	Ledum	Ledum palustre	Wild Rosemary	Respiratory and rheumatic conditions; puncture wounds.

	Abbreviation	Full Name	Common Name	Common Uses
35.	Lycopodium	Lycopodium clavatum	Club Moss	Chronic dyspepsia; pre-examination nerves or stage fright.
36.	Merc Sol.	Mercurius Solubilis	Soluble mercury (quicksilver)	Bad breath; body odour; diarrhoea; chicken pox; mumps.
37.	Nat Mur.	Natrum muriaticum	Sodium Chloride (salt)	Exhaustion; sinus troubles; cold sores; sneezy colds; runny nose.
38.	Nux Vom.	Nux Vomica	Poison Nut	Nervous indigestion; hangover; constipation; itching piles; stomach pain.
39.	Phytolacca	Phytolacca decandra	Phytolacca	Sore throat; mouth ulceration; difficulty in swallowing; shooting and burning pains likened to electric shocks; loss of voice (aphonia).
40.	Plumbum met.	Plumbum metallicum	Lead	Muscle spasms; muscle weakness.
41.	Pulsatilla	Pulsatilla nigricans	Wind flower	Menstrual problems; change of life; shingles; hay fever; headaches; styes.
42.	Rhus Tox.	Rhus Toxicodendron	Poison Ivy	Rheumatism; strains of joints and tendons; lumbago; sciatica; herpes of lips.
43.	Ruta Grav.	Ruta graveolens	Bitterwort	Eyestrain; dislocations and bruised bones; aching and lightness in chest.
44.	Sepia	Sepia officinalis	Cuttlefish (juice)	Change of life; morning sickness; suppressed or delayed periods.

	Abbreviation	Full Name	Common Name	Common Uses
45.	Symphytum	Symphytum officinale	Comfrey	Bone injuries; rheumatic and arthritic conditions resulting from bone fractures.
46.	Silica	Silicea	Pure flint	Boils; abcesses; sinus troubles; chronic headaches.
47.	Sulphur	Sulphur	Sulphur	Skin troubles; boils; burning and itching piles.
48.	Thuja	Thuja occidentalis	Tree of life	Warts; body odour; morning headaches with lack of appetite.
49.	Urtica	Urtica Urens	Stinging nettle	Urticaria; burns and scalds; insect bites; sunburn; gout.
50.	Veratrum alb.	Veratrum album	White Hellebore	Neuralgia; menstrual tension; mental illness.

A-Z List of Homœopathic Medicines

There are over 2,500 homœopathic medicines. As a result of new provings, additions have been made over the years. Some medicines are used very rarely and others are no longer used.

Homœopathic medicines may be freely available in all potencies, but others may only be available in higher potencies or on a doctors' prescription. They may be prescribed in the form of tablets, pilules, granules, powders or liquids.

The main homœopathic medicines are listed. Alternative names, which are commonly used, are also given, and where possible, an indication of the source. Those medicines listed in the 'plant' category may be derived from trees or bark, shrubs, flowers, vegetables, leaves, stems, fruit, berries, roots, bulbs or corms or seeds. 'Mineral' sources may be naturally occurring ores, simple or complex metal salts, acids or alkalis. Organic compounds may be naturally occurring, or rarely of synthetic origin, or extracted from animal or plant matter. Detailed information is given in Homœopathic Pharmacopœia and Homœopathic Materia Medica.

Key to abbreviations (Source)

A	—	Animal
An	—	Antibiotic
An/OC	—	Antibiotic/Organic Compound
E	—	Element
E(M)	—	Element (Metal)
Ess	—	Essence
M	—	Mineral
MA	—	Mineral Acid
MS	—	Marine Sponge
N	—	Nosode
OC	—	Organic Compound
P	—	Plant
R	—	Resin
S	—	Spore
V	—	Vitamin
V/A	—	Vitamin/Animal

A

1. ABELMOSCHUS *P*
2. ABIES CANADENSIS *P*
3. ABIES NIGRA *P*
4. ABIES PECTINATA *P*
5. ABROTANUM (ARTEMISIA ABROTANUM) *P*
6. ABSINTHIUM (ARTEMISIA ABSINTHIUM) *P*
7. ACALYPHA INDICA *P*
8. ACER CAMPESTRE *P*
9. ACER NEGUNDO *P*
10. ACETANILIDUM *OC*

11. ACETICUM ACIDUM
(ACIDUM
ACETICUM) *MA*
12. ACETONUM
(ACETONE) *OC*
13. ACHILLEA
MILLEFOLIUM
(MILLEFOLIUM) *P*
14. ACHILLEA
MOSCHATA *P*
15. ACONITUM
FEROX *P*
16. ACONITUM
NAPELLUS *P*
17. ACORUS
CALAMUS *P*
18. ACTÆA
RACEMOSA *P*
19. ACTÆA SPICATA *P*
20. ADANSONIA
DIGITATA *P*
21. ADEPS SUILLUS *P*
22. ADIANTUM
CAPILLUS
VENERIS *P*
23. ADONIS
VERNALIS *P*
24. ADRENALINUM
(ADRENALIN) *OC*
25. ADULAIRE
26. ÆGOPODIUM
PODAGRARIA *P*
27. ÆSCULUS
GLABRA *P*
28. ÆSCULUS
HIPPOCASTANUM *P*
29. ÆTHIOPS
MERCURIALIS
MINERALIS *M*
30. ÆTHUSA
CYNAPIUM *P*
31. AGARICUS
BULBOSUS *P*
32. AGARICUS
CAMPESTER *P*
33. AGARICUS
MUSCARIUS *P*
34. AGAVE
AMERICANA *P*

35. AGNUS CASTUS *P*
36. AGRAPHIS
NUTANS *P*
37. AGRIMONIA
EUPATORIA *P*
38. AGROPYRUM
REPENS (TRITICUM
REPENS) *P*
39. AILANTHUS
GLANDULOSA *P*
40. AJUGA
CHAMÆPITYS *P*
41. AJUGA REPTANS *P*
42. ALBURNUM
TILIÆ *P*
43. ALCHEMILLA
ALPINA *P*
44. ALCHEMILLA
VULGARIS *P*
45. ALDOSTERONE *OC*
46. ALETRIS FARINOSA *P*
47. ALFALFA *P*
48. ALISMA
PLANTAGO *P*
49. ALLIUM CEPA
(CEPA) *P*
50. ALLIUM PORRUM *P*
51. ALLIUM
SATIVUM *P*
52. ALLIUM
URSINUM *P*
53. ALLOXANUM *OC*
54. ALNUS GLUTINOSA *P*
55. ALOE *P*
56. ALTHÆA
OFFICINALIS *P*
57. ALUMINA
(ALUMINIUM
OXIDE) *M*
58. AMANITA
MUSCARIA (AGARICUS
MUSCARIUS) *P*
59. AMBRA GRISEA *P*
60. AMBROSIA
ARTEMISIÆFOLIA *P*
61. AMMI MAGUS *P*
62. AMMI VISNAGA *P*

63. AMMONIUM
    CARBONICUM *M*
64. AMMONIUM
    MURIATICUM *M*
65. AMMONIUM
    PHOSPHORICUM *M*
66. AMMONIUM
    TARTARICUM *M*
67. AMPELOPSIS
    QUINQUEFOLIA *P*
68. AMPELOPSIS
    WEITCHII *P*
69. AMYGDALES *A*
70. AMYGDALUS
    COMMUNIS
    AMARA *P*
71. AMYGDALUS
    COMMUNIS
    DULCIS *P*
72. AMYGDALUS
    PERSICA (PERSICA
    VULGARIS) *P*
73. AMYLIUM
    NITROSUM *OC*
74. ANACARDIUM
    OCCIDENTALE *P*
75. ANACARDIUM
    ORIENTALE *P*
76. ANAGALLIS
    ARVENSIS *P*
77. ANANASSA
    SATIVA *P*
78. ANANTHERUM
    MURICATUM *P*
79. ANCHUSA
    OFFICINALIS *P*
80. ANEMONE
    PULSATILLA
    (PULSATILLA) *P*
81. ANETHUM
    GRAVEOLENS *P*
82. ANGELICA
    ARCHANGELICA *P*
83. ANGELICA
    SINENSIS RADIX *P*
84. ANGELICA
    SYLVESTRIS *P*
85. ANGUSTURA
    VERA *P*

86. ANISUM
    STELLATUM *P*
87. ANTHEMIS
    NOBILIS *P*
88. ANTHRACINUM
89. ANTHYLLIS
    VULNERARIA *P*
90. ANTIMONIUM
    ARSENICOSUM *M*
91. ANTIMONIUM
    CRUDUM *E*
92. ANTIMONIUM
    IODATUM *M*
93. ANTIMONIUM
    METALLICUM *E(M)*
94. ANTIMONIUM
    SULFURATUM
    AUREUM *M*
95. ANTIMONIUM
    TARTARICUM
    (TARTARUS
    EMETICUS) *M*
96. AORTE *A*
97. APATITE *M*
98. APIS MELLIFICA *A*
99. APIUM DULCE
    (APIUM
    GRAVEOLENS) *P*
100. APIUM VIRUS
     (APISINUM) *P*
101. APOCYNUM
     CANNABINUM *P*
102. AQUA MARINA
103. AQUILEGIA
     VULGARIS *P*
104. ARALIA RACEMOSA *P*
105. ARANEA DIADEMA
106. ARBUTUS
     ANDRACHNE *P*
107. ARBUTUS UNEDO *P*
108. ARCTIUM LAPPA
     (LAPPA MAJOR) *P*
109. ARENARIA RUBRA *P*
110. ARGEMONE
     MEXICANA *P*
111. ARGENT NATIF *M*
112. ARGENTUM
     METALLICUM *E(M)*

113. ARGENTUM NITRICUM *M*
114. ARN
115. ARNICA MONTANA *P*
116. ARSENICUM ALBUM *M*
117. ARSENICUM IODATUM *M*
118. ARSENICUM METALLICUM *E(M)*
119. ARTEMISIA ABROTANUM (ABROTANUM) *P*
120. ARTEMISIA ABSINTHIUM *P*
121. ARTEMISIA CINA (CINA) *P*
122. ARTEMISIA DRACUNCULUS *P*
123. ARTEMISIA MARITIMA (CINA) *P*
124. ARTEMISIA VULGARIS *P*
125. ARTERE *A*
126. ARTERE CORONAIRE *A*
127. ARTERE AORTE (AORTE) *A*
128. ARTERE CORONAIRE *A*
129. ARUM DRACUNCULUS *P*
130. ARUM MACULATUM *P*
131. ARUM TRIPHYLLUM *P*
132. ARUNDO DONAX *P*
133. ASA FŒTIDA *R*
134. ASARUM EUROPÆUM *P*
135. ASCLEPIAS CORNUTI (ASCLEPIAS SYRIACA) *P*
136. ASCLEPIAS CURASSAVICA *P*
137. ASCLEPIAS TUBEROSA *P*
138. ASCLEPIAS VINCETOXICUM *P*
139. ASIMINA TRILOBÀ *P*
140. ASPARAGUS OFFICINALIS *P*
141. ASPERGILLUS BRONCHIALIS *P*
142. ASPERGILLUS NIGER *P*
143. ASPERULA ODORATA *P*
144. ASPIDIUM FILIX MAS *P*

145. ASTACUS FLUVIATILIS *P*
146. ASTERIAS RUBENS *P*
147. ASTRAGALUS EXSCAPUS *P*
148. ASTRAGALUS GLYCYPHYLLOS *P*
149. ATROPA BELLADONNA (BELLADONNA) *P*
150. ATROPINUM *OC*
151. AUCUBA JAPONICA *P*
152. AUREOMYCIN *OC*
153. AURUM IODATUM *M*
154. AURUM METALLICUM *E(M)*
155. AURUM MURIATICUM *M*
156. AURUM MURIATICUM NATRONATUM *M*
157. AVENA SATIVA *P*
158. AVIAIRE
159. AVOINE GERMEE (AVENA SATIVA GERMINATA) *P*
160. AXE CORTICO-HYPOTHALAMIQUE *A*
161. AZURITE *M*

B

162. BADIAGA
163. BALLOTA FŒTIDA *P*
164. BALSAMUM PERUVIANUM *P*
165. BALSAMUM TOLUIFERUM *P*
166. BAMBUSA *P*
167. BAPTISIA TINCTORIA *P*
168. BARBIFLORA (ORTHOSIPHON STAMINEUS) *P*
169. BARBULA SQUARROSA *P*
170. BAROSMA CRENATA *P*
171. BARYTA CARBONICA *M*
172. BARYTA IODATA *M*
173. BARYTA MURIATICA *M*
174. BARYTA SULPHURICA *M*

73

175. BASILICUM (OCIMUM BASILICUM) *P*
176. BEDEGUAR *P*
177. BELLADONNA *P*
178. BELLIS PERENNIS *P*
179. BENZOE
180. BENZOICUM ACIDUM *OC*
181. BENZOLUM *OC*
182. BERBERIS AQUIFOLIUM *P*
183. BERBERIS VULGARIS *P*
184. BETAFITE
185. BETA MARITIMA *P*
186. BETA VULGARIS *P*
187. BETONICA OFFICINALIS *P*
188. BETULA ALBA (BETULA PUBESCENS) *P*
189. BIGNONIA CATALPA *P*
190. BILINUM *A*
191. BISMUTHUM (BISMUTHUM SUBNITRICUM) *M*
192. BISMUTHUM METALLICUM *E(M)*
193. BIXA ORELLANA *P*
194. BLATTA ORIENTALIS *A*
195. BLE GERME *P*
196. BLENDE *M*
197. BŒRHAVIA HIRSUTA *P*
198. BOLDO *P*
199. BORAX *M*
200. BORNITE *M*
201. BORRAGO OFFICINALIS *P*
202. BOTHROPS LANCEOLATUS (LACHESIS LANCEOLATUS) *A*
203. BOVISTA GIGANTEA *P*
204. BRANCA URSINA *P*
205. BRASSICA NAPUS *P*
206. BRASSICA NAPUS OLEIFERA *P*
207. BRASSICA NIGRA *P*
208. BRASSICA OLERACEA *P*

209. BROMUM (BROMIUM) (BROMINE) *E*
210. BRONCHES *A*
211. BRUNELLA VULGARIS *P*
212. BRYONIA (BRYONIA ALBA = BRYONIA DIOICA) *P*
213. BRYOPHYLLUM CALYCINUM *P*
214. BUCHU (BAROSMA CRENATA) *P*
215. BUFO (RANA BUFO)
216. BULBINUM (BULBE RACHIDIEN) *A*
217. BUPLEURUM FALCATUM *P*
218. BURSA PASTORIS (THLASPI BURSA PASTORIS) *P*
219. BUTYRICUM ACIDUM *OC*
220. BUXUS SEMPERVIRENS *P*

C

221. CACAO *P*
222. CACTUS GRANDIFLORUS *P*
223. CACTUS OPUNTIA (OPUNTIA VULGARIS) *P*
224. CADMIUM METALLICUM *E(M)*
225. CADMIUM SULPHURICUM *M*
226. CAJUPUTUM *Ess*
227. CALADIUM SEGUINUM *P*
228. CALAMINTHA GRANDIFLORA *P*
229. CALAMINTHA OFFICINALIS *P*
230. CALCAREA CARBONICA OSTREARUM *M*
231. CALCAREA FLUORICA *M*
232. CALCAREA IODATA *M*

74

233. CALCAREA OSTREICA
(CALCAREA CARBONICA
OSTREARUM) M
234. CALCAREA
PHOSPHORICA M
235. CALCAREA PICRATA M
236. CALCAREA SILICICA M
237. CALCAREA
SULPHURICA M
238. CALCULI BILIARII
239. CALCULI RENALIS
240. CALENDULA
ARVENSIS P
241. CALENDULA
OFFICINALIS P
242. CALLUNA VULGARIS P
243. CALOTROPIS
GIGANTEA P
244. CALTHA PALUSTRIS P
245. CAMPHORA OC
246. CAMPHOROSMA
MONSPELIACUM P
247. CANDIDA ALBICANS
(MONILIA ALBICANS) P
248. CANTHARIS A
249. CAPSELLA BURSA
PASTORIS (THLASPI
BURSA PASTORIS) P
250. CAPSICUM ANNUUM P
251. CARBO ANIMALIS P
252. CARBO VEGETABILIS P
253. CARBOLICUM
ACIDUM MA
254. CARBONEUM
SULPHURATUM M
255. CARDAMINE
PRATENSIS P
256. CARDINE A
257. CARDUUS BENEDICTUS
(CNICUS
BENEDICTUS) P
258. CARDUUS MARIANUS P
259. CARICA PAPAYA P
260. CARLINA ACAULIS P
261. CARLINA VULGARIS P
262. CARPINUS BETULUS P
263. CARTILAGE DE
CONJUGAISON A

264. CARTILAGO
(CARTILAGE) A
265. CARUM CARVI P
266. CARYOPHYLLUS
AROMATICUS (EUGENIA
CARYOPHYLLATA) P
267. CASCARA SAGRADA P
268. CASCARILLA P
269. CASSIA ANGUSTIFOLIA
(SENNA) P
270. CASSIA
OCCIDENTALIS P
271. CASTANEA VESCA P
272. CASTOR EQUI
273. CASTOREUM
274. CAULOPHYLLUM
THALICTROIDES P
275. CAUSTICUM M
276. CEANOTHUS
AMERICANUS P
277. CEDRON P
278. CEDRUS LIBANI P
279. CENCHRIS CONTORTRIX
280. CENTAUREA CYANUS P
281. CENTAUREA NIGRA P
282. CENTELLA ASIATICA
(HYDROCOTYLE
ASIATICA) P
283. CENTRANTHUS
RUBER P
284. CEPHALANDRA
INDICA P
285. CERCIS
SILIQUASTRUM P
286. CEREBELLUM
(CERVELET) A
287. CEREBRINUM
(CEREBRINE =
CERVEAU) A
288. CEREUS BONPLANDII P
289. CEREUS GRANDIFLORUS
(CACTUS
GRANDIFLORUS) P
290. CETRARIA ISLANDICA P
291. CHÆROPHYLLUM
SATIVUM P
292. CHALCOPYRITE M

293. CHAMOMILLA VULGARIS *P*
294. CHEIRANTHUS CHEIRI *P*
295. CHELIDONIUM MAJUS *P*
296. CHELONE GLABRA *P*
297. CHENOPODIUM ANTHELMINTICUM (CHENOPODIUM AMBROSIOIDES) *P*
298. CHIMAPHILIA UMBELLATA *P*
299. CHINA REGIA *P*
300. CHINA RUBRA (CHINA) *P*
301. CHININUM ARSENICOSUM *M*
302. CHININUM SULPHURICUM *M*
303. CHIONANTHUS VIRGINICA *P*
304. CHLORALUM
305. CHLORAMPHENICOLUM (CHLORAMPHENICOL) *OC*
306. CHLOROFORMIUM *OC*
307. CHLORPROMAZINE *OC*
308. CHOLESTERINUM *N*
309. CHRYSANTHEMUM CORONARIUM *P*
310. CHRYSAROBINUM *N*
311. CICER ARIETINUM *P*
312. CICHORIUM INTYBUS *P*
313. CICUTA VIROSA *P*
314. CIMICIFUGA (ACTÆA RACEMOSA) *P*
315. CINA *P*
316. CINCHONA SUCCIRUBRA (CHINA RUBRA) *P*
317. CINERARIA MARITIMA *P*
318. CINNABARIS (MERCURIC SULPHIDE) *M*
319. CINNAMOMUM ZEYLANICUM *P*
320. CIRSIUM ARVENSE *P*
321. CISTUS CANADENSIS *P*
322. CITRUS AURANTIUM *P*

323. CITRUS DECUMANA *P*
324. CITRUS LIMONUM *P*
325. CITRUS VULGARIS *P*
326. CLAVATUM (LYCOPODIUM CLAVATUM) *S*
327. CLEMATIS ERECTA *P*
328. CLEMATIS VITALBA *P*
329. CNICUS BENEDICTUS *P*
330. COBALTUM METALLICUM *E(M)*
331. COCA *P*
332. COCCULUS INDICUS *P*
333. COCCUS CACTI *P*
334. COCHLEARIA ARMORACIA *P*
335. COCHLEARIA OFFICINALIS *P*
336. CŒSIUM MURIATICUM
337. COFFEA CRUDA *P*
338. COFFEA TOSTA *P*
339. COLCHICUM AUTUMNALE
340. COLIBACILLINUM *N*
341. COLLINSONIA CANADENSIS *P*
342. COLOCYNTHIS *P*
343. COLOMBO *P*
344. COLON *A*
345. COLUBRINA (NUX VOMICA) *P*
346. COLUTEA ARBORESCENS *P*
347. COMBRETUM RAIMBAULTI (COMBRETUM MICRANTHUM) *P*
348. CONCHIOLINUM *N*
349. CONDURANGO *P*
350. CONGLOMERAT
351. CONIUM MACULATUM *P*
352. CONVALLARIA MAJALIS *P*
353. CONVOLVULUS ARVENSIS *P*
354. CORALLIUM RUBRUM

355. CORIANDRUM
SATIVUM P
356. CORIARIA
MYRTIFOLIA P
357. CORNUS MAS P
358. CORNUS SANGUINEA P
359. CORPUS LUTEUM
(LUTEINUM) N
360. CORROSIVUS
(MERCURIUS
CORROSIVUS) M
361. CORTEX CEREBRAL A
362. CORTEX SURRENAL
(CORTICO
SURRENALE) A
363. CORTISONE OC
364. CORYDALIS FORMOSA P
365. CORYLUS AVELLANA P
366. CRATÆGUS
OXYACANTHA P
367. CRESOLUM
(CRESOL) OC
368. CROCUS SATIVUS P
369. CROTALUS
HORRIDUS P
370. CROTON TIGLIUM P
371. CUCURBITA MAXIMA P
372. CUCURBITA PEPO P
373. CUMINUM CYMINUM P
374. CUPRESSUS
SEMPERVIRENS P
375. CUPRUM ACETICUM M
376. CUPRUM
ARSENICOSUM M
377. CUPRUM
METALLICUM E
378. CUPRUM OXYDATUM
NIGRUM M
379. CUPRUM
SULPHURICUM M
380. CURARE P
381. CURCUMA (CURCUMA
LONGA = CURCUMA
XANTHORRHIZA) P
382. CYANATUS (MERCURIUS
CYANATUS) M
383. CYANOCOBALAMINE
(VITAMIN B 12) V

384. CYCLAMEN
EUROPEAUM P
385. CYDONIA VULGARIS P
386. CYNARA
CARDUNCULUS P
387. CYNARA SCOLYMUS P
388. CYPRIPEDIUM
PUBESCENS P
389. CYRTOPODIUM P
390. CYSTOSEIRA
FIBROSA
391. CYSTISUS LABURNUM P

D

392. DACTYLIS
GLOMERATA P
393. DAMIANA P
394. DAPHNE MEZEREUM
(MEZEREUM) P
395. DATURA STRAMONIUM
(STRAMONIUM) P
396. DAUCUS CAROTA P
397. DIAPHRAGME A
398. DIENCEPHALE A
399. DIGITALIS PURPUREA P
400. DIOPSIDE
401. DIOSCOREA VILLOSA P
402. DIPHTERICUM N
403. DIPHTEROTOXINUM N
404. DIPLOTAXIS
TENUIFOLIA P
405. DIPSACUS
SYLVESTRIS P
406. DISCI CERVICALES A
407. DISCI LUMBALES A
408. DISCI THORACALES A
409. DOLICHOS
PRURIENS P
410. DROSERA (DROSERA
ROTUNDIFOLIA) P
411. DRYMIS
GRANATENSIS P
412. DRYMIS WINTERI P
413. DULCAMARA P
414. DUODENUM A

E

415. EBERTHINUM   N
416. ECBALLIUM
     ELATERIUM   P
417. ECHINACEA
     ANGUSTIFOLIA   P
418. ELAPS CORALLINUS
419. ENDIVIA SATIVA   P
420. ENTEROCCINUM   N
421. EPHEDRA VULGARIS   P
422. EPIPHYSE   A
423. EQUISETUM ARVENSE   P
424. EQUISETUM
     HÉIMALE   P
425. ERICA CINEREA   P
426. ERICA VULGARIS
     (CALLUNA VULGARIS)   P
427. ERIGERON
     CANADENSIS   P
428. ERIODICTYON
     CALIFORNICUM   P
429. ERUCA SATIVA   P
430. ERYNGIUM
     AQUATICUM   P
431. ERYNGIUM
     CAMPESTRE   P
432. ERYNGIUM
     MARITIMUM   P
433. ERYSIMUM
     OFFICINALE   P
434. ERYTHRÆA
     CENTAURIUM   P
435. ERYTHRINA
     CORALLODENDRON   P
436. ESCHSCHOLTZIA
     CALIFORNICA   P
437. ESTOMAC   A
438. ETHYL SULPHUR
     DICHLORATUM   OC
439. ETHYLICUM (ETHYL
     ALCOHOL)   OC
440. EUCALYPTUS
     GLOBULUS   P
441. EUGENIA
     CARYOPHYLLATA   P
442. EUGENIA JAMBOLANA   P
443. EUGENIA JAMBOSA   P

444. EUPATORIUM
     CANNABINUM   P
445. EUPATORIUM
     PERFOLIATUM   P
446. EUPATORIUM
     PURPUREUM   P
447. EUPHORBIA
     HELIOSCOPIA   P
448. EUPHORBIA
     LATHYRIS   P
449. EUPHORBIA
     PILULIFERA   P
450. EUPHORBIA RESINIFERA
     (EUPHORBIUM)   P
451. EUPHORBIA
     SYLVATICA   P
452. EUPHRASIA
     OFFICINALIS   P
453. EVONYMUS
     ATROPURPUREUS   P
454. EVONYMUS
     EUROPÆUS   P

F

455. FABA VESCA   P
456. FABIANA IMBRICATA   P
457. FAGOPYRUM
     ESCULENTUM   P
458. FAGUS SYLVATICA   P
459. FELSPAR   M
460. FEL TAURI (BILINUM)
     (FEL BOVINUM)   N
461. FERRUM METALLICUM
     (FERRUM
     REDACTUM)   E
462. FERRUM
     MURIATICUM   M
463. FERRUM
     PHOSPHORICUM   M
464. FERRUM PICRICUM   M
465. FERULA COMMUNIS   P
466. FICARIA
     RANUNCULOIDES   P
467. FICUS CARICA   P
468. FICUS RELIGIOSA   P

469. FILIX MAS (ASPIDIUM FILIX MAS)
470. FLAVEINUM (LUTEINUM)   N
471. FLUORICUM ACIDUM   MA
472. FŒNICULUM VULGARE   P
473. FŒNUM GRÆCUM   P
474. FOIE (HEPATINE)   A
475. FOLLICULINUM (ŒSTRONE)   N
476. FORMICA RUFA   A
477. FORMICUM ACIDUM (FORMIC ACID)   OC
478. FRAGARIA VESCA   P
479. FRANCISCEA UNIFLORA   P
480. FRAXINUS AMERICANA   P
481. FRAXINUS EXCELSIOR   P
482. FUCUS CRISPUS   P
483. FUCUS NODOSUS   P
484. FUCUS SERRATUS   P
485. FUCUS VESICULOSUS   P
486. FUMARIA OFFICINALIS   P

G

487. GALANTHUS NIVALIS   P
488. GALEGA OFFICINALIS   P
489. GALENA   M
490. GALEOPSIS LADANUM   P
491. GALEOPSIS OCHROLEUCA   P
492. GALEOPSIS TETRAHIT   P
493. GALIUM APARINE   P
494. GANGLIONS LYMPHATIQUES   A
495. GARNIERITE
496. GASTER GALII   A
497. GASTERASE (ESTOMAC)   A

498. GELSEMIUM SEMPERVIRENS   P
499. GENISTA SCOPARIA   P
500. GENISTA TINCTORIA   P
501. GENTIANA LUTEA   P
502. GENTIANA PURPUREA   P
503. GERANIUM MACULATUM   P
504. GERANIUM ROBERTIANUM   P
505. GEUM MONTANUM   P
506. GEUM URBANUM   P
507. GINGKO BILOBA   P
508. GINSENG   P
509. GLANDES MAMMAIRES (MAMELLINE)   A
510. GLANDE PINEALE (EPIPHYSE)   A
511. GLANDES SURRENALES (SURRENINE)   A
512. GLAUCONIE
513. GLECHOMA HEDERACEA   P
514. GLONOINUM (TRI-NITROGLYCERIN) OC
515. GLUTAMICUM ACIDUM   OC
516. GLYCERINUM   OC
517. GLYCRRHIZA GLABRA   P
518. GNAPHALIUM DIOICUM   P
519. GNAPHALIUM POLYCEPHALUM   P
520. GONOTOXINUM   N
521. GOSSYPIUM ARBOREUM   P
522. GOSSYPIUM HERBACEUM   P
523. GRANATUM (PUNICA GRANATUM)   P
524. GRAPHITES   E
525. GRATIOLA OFFICINALIS   P
526. GRES ROSE
527. GRINDELIA ROBUSTA   P
528. GUACO   P
529. GUAIACUM   P

530. GUARANA (PAULLINIA
SORBILIS) *P*
531. GUMMI
AMMONIACUM *R*

H

532. HALOPERIDOL
533. HAMAMELIS
VIRGINIANA *P*
534. HARPAGOPHYTUM
PROCUMBENS *P*
535. HEDERA HELIX *P*
536. HELIANTHEMUM
VULGARE *P*
537. HELIANTHUS
ANNUUS *P*
538. HELLEBORUS NIGER *P*
539. HELMINTHOCORTON *P*
540. HELONIAS DIOICA *P*
541. HEMATITE *M*
542. HEPAR SULPHUR
(HEPAR SULPHURIS
CALCAREUM) *M*
543. HEPATICA
TRILOBA *P*
544. HEPATINE *A*
545. HERACLEUM
SPHONDYLIUM *P*
546. HERNIARIA GLABRA
(HERNIARIA
VULGARIS) *P*
547. HIERACIUM
PILOSELLA *P*
548. HISTAMINUM *N*
549. HOANG-NAN *P*
550. HOLARRHENA
ANTIDYSENTERICA *P*
551. HORDEUM VULGARE *P*
552. HUMULUS LUPULUS *P*
553. HURA BRASILIENSIS *P*
554. HYDRANGEA
ARBORESCENS *P*
555. HYDRARGYRUM
SULPHURATUM
NIGRUM *P*

556. HYDRASTIS
CANADENSIS *P*
557. HYDROCOTYLE
ASIATICA *P*
558. HYDROCYANICUM
ACIDUM *MA*
559. HYOCYAMUS NIGER *P*
560. HYPERICUM
PERFORATUM *P*
561. HYPOPHYSINE *A*
562. HYPOPHYSINE L.A. *A*
563. HYPOPHYSINE L.P. *A*
564. HYPOTHALAMUS *A*
565. HYSSOPUS
OFFICINALIS *P*

I

566. IAMARA
(IGNATIA AMARA) *P*
567. IBERIS AMARA *P*
568. IGNATIA AMARA *P*
569. ILEX AQUIFOLIUM *P*
570. ILEX PARAGUAYENSIS *P*
571. ILLICIUM ANISATUM
(ANISUM
STELLATUM) *P*
572. INDIGO *OC*
573. INFLUENZINUM *N*
574. INSULINUM *A*
575. INTESTIN GRELE *A*
576. INULA HELENIUM *P*
577. INULA VISCOSA *P*
578. IODUM *E*
579. IPECACUANHA *P*
580. IPOMŒA JALAPA
(JALAPA) *P*
581. IRIDIUM
METALLICUM *E(M)*
582. IRIS TENAX
(IRIS MINOR) *P*
583. IRIS VERSICOLOR *P*

J

584. JABORANDI *P*
585. JACARANDA CAROBA *P*
586. JALAPA *P*
587. JASPE VERT
588. JEQUIRITY *P*
589. JONESIA ASOCA *P*
590. JUGLANS CINEREA *P*
591. JUGLANS REGIA *P*
592. JUNCUS EFFUSUS *P*
593. JUNIPERUS COMMUNIS *P*
594. JUNIPERUS OXYCEDRUS *P*
595. JUSTICIA ADHATODA *P*

K

596. KALIUM ARSENICOSUM *M*
597. KALIUM BICHROMICUM *M*
598. KALIUM BROMATUM *M*
599. KALIUM CARBONICUM *M*
600. KALIUM CHLORICUM *M*
601. KALIUM IODATUM *M*
602. KALIUM MURIATICUM *M*
603. KALIUM NITRICUM *M*
604. KALIUM PHOSPHORICUM *M*
605. KALIUM SULPHURICUM *M*
606. KALMIA LATIFOLIA *P*
607. KAMALA *P*
608. KAWA-KAWA (PIPER METHYSTICUM) *P*
609. KINKELIBA (COMBRETUM RAIMBULTI) *P*

610. KOLA *P*
611. KOUSSO *A*
612. KREOSOTUM *OC*

L

613. LAC CANINUM *A*
614. LAC DEFLORATUM *A*
615. LACHESIS LANCEOLATUS (BOTHROPS LANCEOLATUS)
616. LACHESIS MUTUS (LACHESIS) (LACHESIS MUTA) *A*
617. LACHNANTHES TINCTORIA *P*
618. LACTICUM ACIDUM *OC*
619. LACTUCA SATIVA *P*
620. LACTUCA VIROSA *P*
621. LAMINARIA DIGITATA *P*
622. LAMIUM ALBUM *P*
623. LAMIUM AMPLEXICAULE *P*
624. LAMIUM GALEOBDOLON *P*
625. LAMIUM MACULATUM *P*
626. LAMIUM PURPUREUM *P*
627. LAMPSANA COMMUNIS *P*
628. LAPIS ALBUS
629. LAPPA MAJOR (ARCTIUM LAPPA) *P*
630. LAPPA MINOR *P*
631. LATHYRUS SATIVUS *P*
632. LATRODECTUS MACTANS
633. LAUROCERASUS *P*
634. LAURUS NOBILIS *P*
635. LAVANDULA SPICA *P*
636. LAVANDULA VERA *P*
637. LAZULITE *M*
638. LEDUM PALUSTRE *P*
639. LEMNA GIBBA *P*
640. LEMNA MINOR *P*

641. LEONURUS CARDIACA   *P*
642. LEPIDOLITE   *P*
643. LEPTANDRA
VIRGINICA   *P*
644. LESPEDEZA CAPITATA   *P*
645. LEVISTICUM
OFFICINALE   *P*
646. LEVOMEPROMAZINE   *OC*
647. LIATRIS SPICATA   *P*
648. LIGAMENTS   *A*
649. LIGAMENT
VERTEBRAL   *A*
650. LIGUSTRUM
VULGARE   *P*
651. LILIUM ALBUM   *P*
652. LILIUM TIGRINUM   *P*
653. LIMULUS
654. LINARIA VULGARIS   *P*
655. LINUM
USITATISSIMUM   *P*
656. LITHIUM
CARBONICUM   *M*
657. LITHOSPERMUM
ARVENSE   *P*
658. LITHOSPERMUM
OFFICINALE   *P*
659. LOBELIA CARDINALIS   *P*
660. LOBELIA ERINUS   *P*
661. LOBELIA INFLATA   *P*
662. LOLIUM
TEMULENTUM   *P*
663. LONICERA
CAPRIFOLIUM   *P*
664. LONICERA NIGRA   *P*
665. LOPHOPHYTUM
LEANDRI   *P*
666. LOTUS
CORNICULATUS   *P*
667. LUESINUM   *N*
668. LUPULINUM   *A*
669. LUTEINUM   *A*
670. LYCOPODIUM
CLAVATUM   *P*
671. LYCOPUS EUROPÆUS   *P*
672. LYCOPUS VIRGINICUS   *P*

673. LYSIMACHIA
NUMMULARIA   *P*
674. LYTHRUM SALICARIA   *P*

M

675. MAGNESIA
BOROCITRICA   *M*
676. MAGNESIA
CABONICA   *M*
677. MAGNESIA
MURIATICA   *M*
678. MAGNESIA
PHOSPHORICA   *M*
679. MAGNESIA
SULPHURICA   *M*
680. MAGNESIUM
METALLICUM   *E(M)*
681. MAGNOLIA
GRANDIFLORA   *P*
682. MAHONIA AQUIFOLIUM
(BERBERIS
AQUIFOLIUM)   *P*
683. MALUS COMMUNIS   *P*
684. MALVA MOSCHATA   *P*
685. MALVA SYLVESTRIS   *P*
686. MAMELLINE   *A*
687. MANDRAGORA
OFFICINARUM   *P*
688. MANGANUM
ACETICUM   *M*
689. MANGANUM
METALLICUM   *E(M)*
690. MARBRE SACCHAROIDE
691. MARRUBIUM
VULGARE   *P*
692. MATICO   *P*
693. MATRICARIA
CHAMOMILLA
(CHAMOMILLA
VULGARIS)   *P*
694. MEDICAGO SATIVA
(ALFALFA)   *P*
695. MEDORRHINUM
(GONOCOCCIN)   *N*

696. MEDULLINE *A*
697. MEDULLO-
    SURRENALE *A*
678. MEDULOSS *A*
699. MELILOTUS
    OFFICINALIS *P*
700. MELISSA OFFICINALIS *P*
701. MELITTIS
    MELISSOPHYLLUM *P*
702. MENADIONE
    (VITAMIN K3) *V/A*
703. MENTHA ARVENSIS *P*
704. MENTHA PIPERITA *P*
705. MENTHA PULEGIUM *P*
706. MENTHA
    ROTUNDIFOLIA *P*
707. MENTHA SYLVESTRIS *P*
708. MENTHA VIRIDIS *P*
709. MENYANTHES
    TRIFOLIATA *P*
710. MEPHITIS PUTORIUS
711. MERCURIALIS ANNUA *P*
712. MERCURIALIS
    PERENNIS *P*
713. MERCURIUS
    (MERCURIUS VIVUS) *M*
714. MERCURIUS
    BI-IODATUS *M*
715. MERCURIUS
    CORROSIVUS *M*
716. MERCURIUS
    CYANATUS *M*
717. MERCURIUS DULCIS *M*
718. MERCURIUS
    PROTO-IODATUS
    (MERCURIUS
    IODATUS) *M*
719. MERCURIUS
    SOLUBILIS *M*
720. MERCURIUS VIVUS *M*
721. METALDEHYDUM *OC*
722. METALLUM ALBUM
    (ARSENICUM ALBUM) *M*
723. METALLUM IODATUM
    (ARSENICUM
    IODATUM) *M*
724. METHYSERGIDE
725. MEZEREUM *P*

726. MILLEFOLIUM
    (ACHILLEA
    MILLEFOLIUM) *P*
727. MIRABILIS JALAPA *P*
728. MŒLLE EPINIERE
    (MEDULLINE) *A*
729. MŒLLE OSSEUSE
    (MEDULOSS) *A*
730. MOMORDICA
    BALSAMINA *P*
731. MONAZITE
732. MONILIA ALBICANS *P*
733. MORBILLINUM *N*
734. MORUS NIGRA *P*
735. MOSCHUS *P*
736. MUCOR MUCEDO *P*
737. MUIRA PUAMA *P*
738. MUQUEUSE ANALE *A*
739. MUQUEUSE DU COLON
    (COLON) *A*
740. MUQUEUSE DUODENALE
    (DUODENUM) *A*
741. MUQUEUSE GASTRIQUE
    (ESTOMAC) *A*
742. MUQUEUSE NASALE
    (MUQUEUSE
    ENDONASALE) *A*
743. MUQUEUSE
    RHINO-PHARYNGEE *A*
744. MUQUEUSE
    SINUSALE *A*
745. MUQUEUSE STOMACALE
    (ESTOMAC) *A*
746. MUQUEUSE UTERINE
    (UTERINE) *A*
747. MUREX PURPUREA
748. MURIATICUM
    ACIDUM *MA*
749. MUSCLE LISSE *A*
750. MUSCLE STRIE *A*
751. MYOCARDE
    (CARDINE) *A*
752. MYOSOTIS ARVENSIS *P*
753. MYRICA CERIFERA *P*
754. MYRISTICA SEBIFERA *P*
755. MYRRH (MYRRHA) *R*
756. MYRRHIS ODORATA *P*
757. MYRTUS COMMUNIS *P*

N

758. NAJA TRIPUDIANS
759. NAPHTALINUM *OC*
760. NASTURTIUM OFFICINALE *P*
761. NATRUM CARBONICUM *M*
762. NATRUM CHLORICUM *M*
763. NATRUM MURIATICUM *M*
764. NATRUM PHOSPHORICUM *M*
765. NATRUM SULPHURICUM *M*
766. NEPENTHES *P*
767. NEPETA CATARIA *P*
768. NEPHRINE (RENINE) *A*
769. NERFS *A*
770. NERF OCCIPITAL *A*
771. NERIUM OLEANDER *P*
772. NICCOLUM METALLICUM *E(M)*
773. NICOTIANA TABACUM (TABACUM) *P*
774. NIGELLA DAMASCENA *P*
775. NIGELLA SATIVA *P*
776. NITRICUM ACIDUM (NITRIC ACID) *MA*
777. NUX MOSCHATA *P*
778. NUX VOMICA *P*
779. NYCTERINIA CAPENSIS *P*
780. NYMPHÆA ALBA *P*
781. NYMPHÆA LUTEA *P*

O

782. OBSIDIENNE
783. OCIMUM BASILICUM *P*
784. OCIMUM CANUM *P*
785. ŒNANTHE CROCATA *P*
786. ŒNANTHE PHELLANDRIUM *P*

787. ŒNOTHERA BIENNIS *P*
788. OLEA EUROPÆA *P*
789. OLEANDER (NERIUM OLEANDER) *P*
790. OLIBANUM *R*
791. ONONIS REPENS *P*
792. ONONIS SPINOSA *P*
793. ONOSMODIUM VIRGINIANUM *P*
794. OPIUM *P*
795. OPUNTIA VULGARIS *P*
796. ORCHITINUM *N*
797. ORGE GERMEE *P*
798. ORIGANUM MAJORANA *P*
799. ORIGANUM VULGARE *P*
800. OR NATIF (AURUM METALLICUM) *E(M)*
801. ORNITHOGALUM UMBELLATUM *P*
802. ORPIMENT
803. ORTHOSIPHON STAMINEUS *P*
804. OSMUNDA REGALIS *P*
805. OSSEINE (OSSEINUM) *A*
806. OVARINUM (OVAIRE) *A*
807. OXALICUM ACIDUM *OC*
808. OXYDENDRUM ARBOREUM *P*
809. OXYURUS VERMICULARIS *P*

P

810. PÆONIA OFFICINALIS *P*
811. PALIURUS ACULEATUS (PALIURUS AUSTRALIS) *P*
812. PALLADIUM METALLICUM *E(M)*
813. PANCREINE (PANCREAS) *A*
814. PAPAVER RHŒAS *P*

815. PARATHYROIDINUM *N*
816. PARATHYROIDINUM B *N*
817. PAREIRA BRAVA *P*
818. PARIETARIA OFFICINALIS *P*
819. PARIS QUADRIFOLIA *P*
820. PARNASSIA PALUSTRIS *P*
821. PAROI ARTERIELLE (ARTERE) *A*
822. PAROTIDINUM (PAROTIDINE) *P*
823. PASSIFLORA INCARNATA *P*
824. PAULLINIA SORBILIS (GUARANA) *P*
825. PEAU *A*
826. PELARGONIUM ODORATISSIMUM *P*
827. PENICILLINUM *An/OC*
828. PENICILLIUM CANDIDUM *An/OC*
829. PENICILLIUM NOTATUM *An/OC*
830. PERHEXILLINE
831. PERSEA GRATISSMA *P*
832. PERSICA VULGARIS *P*
833. PERTUSSINUM *N*
834. PETASITES FRAGRANS (TUSSILAGO FRAGRANS) *P*
835. PETASITES OFFICINALIS *P*
836. PETROLEUM *OC*
837. PETROSELINUM CRISPUM *P*
838. PETROSELINUM SATIVUM *P*
839. PHARYNX *A*
840. PHASEOLUS VULGARIS *OC*
841. PHENOBARBITAL (PHENOBARBITONUM)
842. PHLEUM PRATENSE *P*
843. PHOSPHORICUM ACIDUM *MA*
844. PHOSPHORUS *E*

845. PHOSPHORUS TRI-IODATUS *M*
846. PHRAGMITES COMMUNIS *P*
847. PHYLLANTHUS NIRURI *P*
848. PHYSALIS ALKEKENGI *P*
849. PHYSOSTIGMA VENENOSUM *P*
850. PHYTOLACCA DECANDRA *P*
851. PICRICUM ACIDUM *OC*
852. PILOCARPUS JABORANDI (JABORANDI) *P*
853. PILOSELLA (HIERACIUM PILOSELLA) *P*
854. PIMPINELLA ANISUM *P*
855. PIMPINELLA SAXIFRAGA *P*
856. PINUS MONTANA *P*
857. PINUS SYLVESTRIS *P*
858. PIPER ANGUSTIFOLIUM (MATICO) *P*
859. PIPER METHYSTICUM *P*
860. PISCIDIA ERYTHRINA *P*
861. PIX LIQUIDA *P*
862. PLACENTINE (PLACENTA) *A*
863. PLANTAGO LANCEOLATA *P*
864. PLANTAGO MAJOR *P*
865. PLANTAGO PSYLLIUM *P*
866. PLATANUS *P*
867. PLATINUM METALLICUM *E(M)*
868. PLEXUS SOLAIRE
869. PLUMBAGO EUROPÆA *P*
870. PLUMBUM IODATUM *M*
871. PLUMBUM METALLICUM *E(M)*
872. PLUMERIA ALBA *P*
873. PODOPHYLLIN *R*
874. PODOPHYLLUM PELTATUM *P*
875. POLLENS (POLLANTINUM)

876. POLONIUM
METALLICUM *E(M)*
877. POLYGALA SENEGA
(SENEGA) *P*
878. POLYGONATUM
VULGARE *P*
879. POLYGONUM
AVICULARE *P*
880. POLYGONUM
BISTORTA *P*
881. POLYGONUM
FAGOPYRUM
(FAGOPYRUM
ESCULENTUM) *P*
882. POLYGONUM
HYDROPIPER *P*
883. POLYPODIUM
VULGARE *P*
884. POLYTRICHUM
COMMUNE *P*
885. POPULUS CANDICANS *P*
886. POPULUS NIGRA *P*
887. POPULUS TREMULA *P*
888. POTENTILLA
ANSERINA *P*
889. POTENTILLA
REPTANS *P*
890. POTENTILLA
TORMENTILLA *P*
891. POTERIUM
SANGUISORBA *P*
892. POTHOS FŒTIDUS *P*
893. POUMON (PULMINE) *A*
894. POUMON HISTAMINE *A*
895. PRIMULA OBCONICA *P*
896. PRIMULA
OFFICINALIS *P*
897. PROGESTERONUM *A*
898. PROLAN (HYPOPHYSINE
L.A.) *A*
899. PROPOLIS
900. PROSTATE
(PROSTATINUM) *A*
901. PROTEUS VULGARIS *P*
902. PRUNUS AMYGDALUS
(AMYGDALUS
COMMUNIS
"DULCIS") *P*

903. PRUNUS LAUROCERASUS
(LAUROCERASUS) *P*
904. PRUNUS SPINOSA *P*
905. PSORINUM *N*
906. PTELEA TRIFOLIATA *P*
907. PULMINE (POUMON) *A*
908. PULMONARIA
OFFICINALIS *P*
909. PULSATILLA (ANEMONE
PULSATILLA = A.
PRATENSIS =
P. NIGRICANS) *P*
910. PUNICA GRANATUM *P*
911. PUTRESCINUM *N*
912. PYRETHRUM
(PYRETHRUM
PARTHENIUM) *P*
913. PYRITES *M*
914. PYROGENIUM
915. PYROLUSITE

Q

916. QUASSIA AMARA *P*
917. QUEBRACHO *P*
918. QUERCUS GLANDIUM *P*
919. QUERCUS
PEDONCULATA *P*
920. QUERCUS ROBUR *P*
921. QUILLAIA SAPONARIA
(SAPONARIA) *P*

R

922. RADIUM
BROMATUM *M*
923. RADIX (IPECA) *P*
924. RANA BUFO
925. RANUNCULUS ACRIS *P*
926. RANUNCULUS
BULBOSUS *P*
927. RANUNCULUS
SCELERATUS *P*

928. RAPHANUS SATIVUS
NIGER *P*
929. RATANHIA *P*
930. RATE (SPLENINE) *A*
931. RAUWOLFIA
SERPENTINA *P*
932. REIN (CORTEX) *A*
933. REIN (MEDULLAIRE) *A*
934. RENINE (REIN) *A*
935. RHAMNUS
CATHARTICA *P*
936. RHAMNUS FRANGULA *P*
937. RHAMNUS ZIZYPHUS *P*
938. RHEUM
OFFICINALE *P*
939. RHODODENDRON
CHRYSANTHUM *P*
940. RHODODENDRON
FERRUGINEUM *P*
941. RHODONITE
942. RHUS AROMATICA *P*
943. RHUS GLABRA *P*
944. RHUS
TOXICODENDRON *P*
945. RHUS VERNIX (RHUS
VENENATA) *P*
946. RIBES NIGRUM *P*
947. RIBES RUBRUM *P*
948. RICINUS COMMUNIS *P*
949. ROBINIA
PSEUDO-ACACIA *P*
950. ROSA CANINA *P*
951. ROSA GALLICA *P*
952. ROSMARINUS
OFFICINALIS *P*
953. RUBIA TINCTORIA *P*
954. RUBUS FRUTICOSUS *P*
955. RUBUS IDÆUS *P*
956. RUMEX ACETOSELLA *P*
957. RUMEX ALPINUS *P*
958. RUMEX AQUATICUS *P*
959. RUMEX CRISPUS *P*
960. RUMEX PATIENTIA *P*
961. RUSCUS ACULEATUS *P*
962. RUTA GRAVEOLENS *P*

S

963. SABADILLA
OFFICINARUM *P*
964. SABAL SERRULATA *P*
965. SABINA *P*
966. SACCHARUM LACTIS *OC*
967. SALICYLICUM
ACIDUM *OC*
968. SALIX ALBA *P*
969. SALIX NIGRICANS *P*
970. SALVIA OFFICINALIS *P*
971. SALVIA PRATENSIS *P*
972. SALVIA SCLAREA *P*
973. SAMBUCUS EBULUS *P*
974. SAMBUCUS NIGRA *P*
975. SANGUINARIA
CANADENSIS *P*
976. SANGUINARINA
NITRICA *P*
977. SANGUISORBA
OFFICINALIS *P*
978. SANICULA EUROPÆA *P*
979. SANTOLINA
CHAMÆCYPARISSUS *P*
980. SAPONARIA
OFFICINALIS *P*
981. SAPOTA ACHRAS *P*
982. SARCOLACTICUM
ACIDUM *OC*
983. SARRACENIA
PURPUREA *P*
984. SARSAPARILLA *P*
985. SASSAFRAS
OFFICINALE *P*
986. SATUREIA
HORTENSIS *P*
987. SATUREIA MONTANA *P*
988. SAXIFRAGA
GRANULATA *P*
989. SCAMMONIUM *P*
990. SCHINUS MOLLE *P*
991. SCILLA BIFOLIA *P*
992. SCILLA MARITIMA *P*
993. SCOLOPENDRIUM
OFFICINALE *P*

994. SCROFULARIA NODOSA *P*
995. SCUTELLARIA GALERICULATA *P*
996. SCUTELLARIA LATERIFLORA *P*
997. SECALE CEREALE *P*
998. SECALE CORNUTUM *P*
999. SEDUM ACRE *P*
1000. SELENIUM METALLICUM *E(M)*
1001. SEMPERVIVUM TECTORUM *P*
1002. SENECIO CORDATUS *P*
1003. SENECIO DORONICUM *P*
1004. SENECIO FUCHSII *P*
1005. SENECIO JACOBÆA *P*
1006. SENECIO SYLVATICUS *P*
1007. SENECIO VULGARIS *P*
1008. SENEGA *P*
1009. SENNA *P*
1010. SEPIA OFFICINALIS *A*
1011. SEQUOIA GIGANTEA *P*
1012. SERRATULA TINCTORIA *P*
1013. SERUM D'ANGUILLE
1014. SERUM ANTICOLIBACILLAIRE
1015. SERUM EQUILINUM
1016. SERUM DE YERSIN
1017. SEVE DE BOULEAU
1018. SIEGESBECKIA ORIENTALIS *P*
1019. SILICEA *M*
1020. SIMARUBA OFFICINALIS *P*
1021. SINAPIS NIGRA (BRASSICA NIGRA) *P*
1022. SINUS (MUQUEUSE SINUSALE) *A*
1023. SMILAX MEDICA (SARSPARILLA) *P*
1024. SOJA HISPIDA *P*
1025. SOLANUM CAROLINENSE *P*
1026. SOLANUM DULCAMARA (DULCAMARA) *P*
1027. SOLANUM LYCOPERSICUM *P*
1028. SOLANUM MALACOXYLON *P*
1029. SOLANUM MELONGENA *P*
1030. SOLANUM NIGRUM *P*
1031. SOLANUM TUBEROSUM *P*
1032. SOLIDAGO VIRGA AUREA *P*
1033. SOLUBILIS (MERCURIUS SOLUBILIS) *M*
1034. SORBUS DOMESTICA *P*
1035. SPARTIUM JUNCEUM *P*
1036. SPIGELIA ANTHELMIA *P*
1037. SPINACIA OLERACEA *P*
1038. SPIRÆA ULMARIA *P*
1039. SPIRITUS QUERCUS GLANDIUM
1040. SPLENINE *A*
1041. SPONGIA TOSTA *MS*
1042. STACHYS ARVENSIS *P*
1043. STACHYS PALUSTRIS *P*
1044. STACHYS SYLVATICA *P*
1045. STANNUM METALLICUM *E(M)*
1046. STAPHYLOCOCCINUM *N*
1047. STAPHYLOTOXINUM *N*
1048. STAPHYSAGRIA *P*
1049. STIBINE
1050. STICTA PULMONARIA *P*
1051. STILLINGIA SYLVATICA *P*
1052. STRAMONIUM *P*
1053. STREPTOCOCCINUM *N*
1054. STREPTOMYCINUM (STREPTOMYCIN) *An*
1055. STRONTIUM CARBONICUM *M*
1056. STRONTIUM IODATUM *M*
1057. STRONTIUM OXYDATUM *M*

1058. STROPHANTHUS HISPIDUS *P*
1059. STRYCHNINUM (STRYCHNINE) *OC*
1060. SUCCINICUM ACIDUM *OC*
1061. SULPHUR (SULFUR) *E*
1062. SULPHUR IODATUM (SULFUR IODATUM) *M*
1063. SULPHURICUM ACIDUM (SULPHURIC ACID) *MA*
1064. SUMBUL (SUMBULUS MOSCHATUS) *P*
1065. SURRENINE (SURRENALES) *A*
1066. SYMPHORICARPUS RACEMOSUS *P*
1067. SYMPHYTUM OFFICINALE *P*
1068. SYRINGA VULGARIS *P*
1069. SYZYGIUM JAMBOLANUM (EUGENIA JAMBOLANA) *P*

T

1070. TABACUM *P*
1071. TABERNANTHE IBOGA *P*
1072. TAMARIX GALLICA *P*
1073. TAMUS COMMUNIS. *P*
1074. TANACETUM BALSAMITA *P*
1075. TANACETUM VULGARE *P*
1076. TARAXACUM DENS LEONIS *P*
1077. TARENTULA HISPANICA *A*
1078. TAXUS BACCATA *P*
1079. TELLURIUM METALLICUM *E(M)*
1080. TENDON *A*
1081. TEREBINTHINA
1082. TESKRA *P*

1083. TESTOSTERONE ACETATE *OC*
1084. TESTOSTERONE PROPIONATE *OC*
1085. TEUCRIUM BOTRYS *P*
1086. TEUCRIUM CHAMÆDRYS *P*
1087. TEUCRIUM MARUM VERUM *P*
1088. TEUCRIUM SCORDIUM *P*
1089. TEUCRIUM SCORODONIA *P*
1090. THALAMUS *A*
1091. THALLIUM ACETICUM *M*
1092. THALLIUM METALLICUM *E(M)*
1093. THALLIUM SULPHURATUM *M*
1094. THEOBROMA CACAO (CACAO) *P*
1095. THERIDION CURRASSAVICUM
1096. THIOPROPERAZINE *OC*
1097. THIOSINAMINUM *OC*
1098. THLASPI BURSA PASTORIS *P*
1099. THUYA OCCIDENTALIS *P*
1100. THYMUS SERPYLLUM *P*
1101. THYMUS VULGARIS *P*
1102. THYMUSINUM (THYMUSINE = THYMUS) *A*
1103. THYROIDEA (THYROIDINUM = THYROID) *A*
1104. TILIA ARGENTEA (TILIA TOMENTOSA) *P*
1105. TILIA EUROPÆA (TILIA CORDATA = TILIA SYLVESTRIS) *P*
1106. TILIÆ ALBURNUM (ALBURNUM TILIÆ) *P*
1107. TISSUE CAPILLAIRE *A*
1108. TISSUE CONJONCTIF *A*
1109. TŒNIA SAGINATA

1110. TOURMALINE LITHIQUE
1111. TRACHYTE
1112. TRAGOPOGON PRATENSIS *P*
1113. TRIFOLIUM PRATENSE *P*
1114. TRIFOLIUM REPENS *P*
1115. TRILLIUM PENDULUM *P*
1116. TRITICUM GERMINATUM *P*
1117. TRITICUM REPENS *P*
1118. TRITICUM VULGARE *P*
1119. TROPÆOLUM MAJUS
1120. T.S.H. (THYREOSTIMULINE HYPOPHYSAIRE)
1121. TUBERCULINUM *N*
1122. TUBERCULINUM RESIDUUM *N*
1123. TUSSILAGO FARFARA *P*
1124. TUSSILAGO FRAGRANS *P*

U

1125. ULEXITE (CALCIUM SODIUM BORATE) *M*
1126. ULMUS CAMPESTRIS *P*
1127. URANIUM NITRICUM *M*
1128. UREA *OC*
1129. URICUM ACIDUM *OC*
1130. URTICA DIOICA *P*
1131. URTICA URENS *P*
1132. USNEA BARBATA *P*
1133. USTILAGO MAIDIS *P*
1134. UTERINE (UTERUS) *A*
1135. UVA URSI *P*

V

1136. VACCINIUM MYRTILLUS *P*
1137. VACCINIUM VITIS IDÆA *P*
1138. VACCINOTOXINUM *N*
1139. VALERIANA OFFICINALIS *P*
1140. VANADIUM METALLICUM *E(M)*
1141. VANILLA PLANIFOLIA *P*
1142. VEIN *A*
1143. VERATRUM ALBUM *P*
1144. VERATRUM VIRIDE *P*
1145. VERBASCUM THAPSUS *P*
1146. VERBENA OFFICINALIS *P*
1147. VERONICA OFFICINALIS *P*
1148. VERTEBRA *A*
1149. VERTEBRE CERVICALE *A*
1150. VERTEBRE DORSALE *A*
1151. VERTEBRE LOMBAIRE *A*
1152. VERTEBRES SACREES *A*
1153. VESICULE BILIAIRE *A*
1154. VESSIE *A*
1155. VIBURNUM LANTANA *P*
1156. VIBURNUM OPULUS *P*
1157. VIBURNUM PRUNIFOLIUM *P*
1158. VICIA FABA (FABA VESCA) *P*
1159. VINCA MAJOR *P*
1160. VINCA MINOR *P*
1161. VINCA ROSEA *P*
1162. VINCETOXICUM OFFICINALE (ASCLEPIAS VINCETOXICUM) *P*
1163. VIOLA ODORATA *P*
1164. VIOLA TRICOLOR *P*
1165. VIPERA REDI (ITALIAN VIPER) *A*

1166. VIPERA TORVA
(GERMAN VIPER) *A*
1167. VISCUM ABIETIS *P*
1168. VISCUM ALBUM *P*
1169. VISCUM CRATÆGI *P*
1170. VISCUM MALI *P*
1171. VISCUM PINI *P*
1172. VISCUM QUERCUS *P*
1173. VITAMIN A
(RETINOL) *V/A*
1174. VITAMIN B1 *V/A*
1175. VITAMIN B2 *V/A*
1176. VITAMIN B6 *V/A*
1177. VITAMIN B12
(CYANOCOBALAMIN) *V/A*
1178. VITAMIN C *V/A*
1179. VITAMIN D2
(CALCIFEROL) *V/A*
1180. VITAMIN D3
(VIGANTOL) *V/A*
1181. VITAMIN E
(∝ – TOCOPHEROL) *V/A*
1182. VITAMIN F
(LINACIDIN) *V/A*
1183. VITAMIN K3
(MENADIONE) *V/A*
1184. VITAMIN P *V/A*
1185. VITAMIN PP *V/A*
1186. VITEX AGNUS CASTUS
(AGNUS CASTUS) *P*
1187. VITIS VINIFERA *P*

W

1188. WHEAT GLUTEN *P*

X

1189. XANTHIUM
MACROCARPUM *P*
1190. XANTHIUM
SPINOSUM *P*
1191. XANTHIUM
STRUMARIUM *P*
1192. X-RAY

Y

1193. YAGE *P*
1194. YERBA SANTA
(ERIODICTYON
CALIFORNICUM) *P*
1195. YOHIMBEHE *P*
1196. YUCCA
FILAMENTOSA *P*

Z

1197. ZEA MAIDIS (STIGMATA
MAIDIS) *P*
1198. ZINCUM
METALLICUM *E(M)*
1199. ZINCUM
PHOSPHORICUM *OC*
1200. ZINCUM
VALERIANICUM *OC*
1201. ZINGIBER
OFFICINALE *P*
1202. ZIZIA AUREA
(THASPIUM AUREM) *P*
1203. ZIZYPHUS JUJUBA *P*

Addresses of National Organisations

The Faculty of Homœopathy

The Royal Homœopathic
Hospital
Great Ormond Street
London WC1N 3HR

**The British Association of
Homœopathic Pharmacists**

Suite 1
19A Cavendish Square
London W1M 9AD

The Hahnemann Society

The Humane Education Centre
Avenue Lodge
Bounds Green Road
London N22 4EU

The Society of Homœopaths

101 Sebastian Avenue
Shenfield
Brentwood
Essex CM15 8PP

**The British Homœopathic
Association**

27A Devonshire Street
London W1N 1RJ

**The Hahnemann College
of Homœopathy**

243 The Broadway
Southall
Middlesex UB1 1NF

**The Homœopathic
Development Foundation**

19A Cavendish Square
London W1M 9AD

**The Homœopathic Trust
for Research and Education**

Hahnemann House
2 Powis Place
Great Ormond Street
London WC1N 3HT

**The National Association
of Homœopathic Groups**

Easter Cottage
School Lane
Middleton Stoney
Oxon

**The British Association
of Homœopathic Veterinary
Surgeons**

Chinham House
Stanford in the Vale
Faringdon Oxon SN7 8NQ

**The British Homœopathy
Research Group**

27 Wimpole Street,
London W1M 7AD

**The Institute for
Complementary Medicine**

21 Portland Place
London W1N 3AF

Bibliography

HAEHL, Richard. *Samuel Hahnemann, His Life and Work* Leipzig, 1922

HAHNEMANN, Samuel. *The Chronic Diseases, Their Peculiar Nature and Their Homœopathic Cure* (translated by Prof. L. H. Tafel from the second German edition, 1835); Boericke and Tafel, Philadelphia, 1896.

HAHNEMANN, Samuel. *Materia Medica Pura Volumes I and II* Hahnemann Publishing Company, 1881.

HAHNEMANN, Samuel. *Organon of the Rational Art of Healing* (translated by C. E. Wheeler from the German edition of 1810) J. M. Dent, 1913.

COOK, Trevor M. *Samuel Hahnemann, Founder of Homœopathy* Thorsons Publishers, 1981.

KNERR, Calvin B. *Life of Hering* Magee Press, 1940.

MITCHELL, G. Ruthven. *Homœopathy* W. H. Allen, 1975.

GORDON-ROSS, A. C. *Homœopathic Green Medicine* Thorsons Publishers, 1978.

POLUNIN, Oleg. *Flowers of Europe* Oxford University Press, 1969.

BOERICKE, W. *Materia Medica with Repertory* Boericke and Runyon, Philadelphia.

CLARKE, J. H. *Clinical Repertory* C. W. Daniel.

KENT, J. T. *Repertory of Homœopathic Materia Medica*

PRATT, N. J. *Homœopathic Prescribing* Beaconsfield Publishers.

The Homœopathic Handbook; Wigmore Publications.

The British Homœopathic Journal; Vol LIX, No 1, 1970.
Ibid.   Vol LIV, No 2, 1965
Ibid.   Vol LX, No 4, 1971
Ibid.   Vol LII, No 4, 1963
Ibid.   Vol LI, No 4, 1962
Ibid.   Vol LIII, No 3, 1964
Ibid.   Vol LVII, No 2, 1968
Ibid.   Vol LXI, No 4, 1972
Ibid.   Vol LV, No 2, 1966
Ibid.   Vol LIII, No 4, 1964
Ibid.   Vol 73, No 3, 1984

DAY, Christopher. *The Homœpathic Treatment of Small Animals* Wigmore
Publications, 1984.